The
Mental
Status Exam

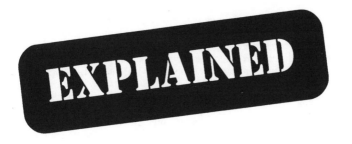

EXPLAINED

David J. Rob
Diplomate
Psych

D1214813

Rapid Psychler Press

Suite 374
3560 Pine Grove Ave.
Port Huron, Michigan
USA 48060

Suite 203
1673 Richmond St.
London, Ontario
Canada N6G 2N3

Toll Free Phone   888-PSY-CHLE (888-779-2453)
Toll Free Fax   888-PSY-CHLR (888-779-2457)
Outside the U.S. & Canada — Fax 519-675-0610
website www.psychler.com
email   rapid@psychler.com

ISBN 1-894328-20-5
Printed in the United States of America
© 2000, Rapid Psychler Press
First Edition, First Printing

All caricatures are purely fictitious. Any resemblance to real people, either living or deceased, is entirely coincidental (and unfortunate). The author assumes no responsibility for the consequences of diagnoses made, or treatment instituted, as a result of the contents of this book – such determinations should be made by qualified mental health professionals. Every effort was made to ensure that the information in this book was accurate at the time of publication. However, due to the changing nature of the field of psychiatry, the reader is encouraged to consult additional and more recent sources of information.

Dedication

This book is dedicated to my secretary
Susan Fletcher

Acknowledgments

I am indebted to the following individuals for their unfailing support in assisting me with this text.

- **Brian & Fanny Chapman**
- **Monty & Lil Robinson**
- **Lisa & Cathy Burgard**
- **Nicole & Mark Kennedy**
- **Dr. Donna Robinson & Dr. Robert Bauer**
- **Dean Avola**
- **Brad Groshok**

I would also like to thank the following people for their helpful reviews of this manuscript.

- **Tom Norry, B.Sc.N.**
- **Jessica Baugniet, M.D.**
- **Lisa & Cathy Burgard**
- **Dr. Sandra Northcott**
- **Dr. Lisa Bogue**
- **Dr. Michelle Kelly**

Rapid Psychler Press

produces books and presentation media that are:
• comprehensively researched
• well organized
• formatted for ease of use
• reasonably priced
• clinically oriented, and
• include humor that enhances education, and that neither demeans patients nor the efforts of those who treat them

Table of Contents

Publication Notes

Terminology
Throughout this book, the term "patient" refers to people who are suffering and seek help. The term further describes those who bear pain without complaint or anger. The terms "consumer" or "consumer-survivor" reflect an unfortunate trend that is pejorative towards mental health care, labeling it as if it were a trade or business instead of a profession. These terms are also ambiguous, as it is not clear what is being "consumed" or "survived."

Graphics
All of the illustrations in this book are original works of art commissioned by Rapid Psychler Press and are a signature feature of our publications. Rapid Psychler Press makes available an entire library of color illustrations (including those from this book) as 35mm slides and overhead transparencies. These images are available for viewing and can be purchased from our website — **www.psychler.com**

These images from our color library may be used for presentations. We request that you respect our copyright and do not reproduce these images in any form for any purpose at any time.

Bolded Terms
Throughout this book, various terms appear in bolded text which allows for ease of identification. Most of these terms are defined in this text. Some, however, are only mentioned because a detailed description is beyond the scope of this book. Fuller explanations of all of the bolded terms can be found in standard reference texts.

1/ Introduction to the Mental Status Exam

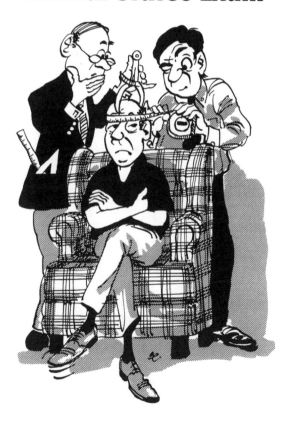

What is the Mental Status Examination?

The **Mental Status Examination (MSE)** is the component of an interview where cognitive functions are tested and inquiries are made about the symptoms of psychiatric conditions. It is a set of standardized observations and questions designed to evaluate:

- **Sensorium**
- **Perception**
- **Thinking**
- **Feeling**
- **Behavior**

The MSE is an integral part of any clinical interview, not just one that takes place in a psychiatric context. An assessment of cognitive functioning must be made before information from patients can be considered reliable and accurate. The MSE records only observed behavior, cognitive abilities, and inner experiences expressed during the interview. It is conducted to assess as completely as possible the factors necessary to arrive at a preferred diagnosis, formulate a treatment plan, and follow a patient's clinical course.

The MSE is a portable assessment tool that helps identify psychiatric symptoms and gauge their severity. With experience, it is a specific, sensitive, and inexpensive diagnostic instrument. The MSE takes only a few minutes to administer yet yields information that is crucial to making a diagnostic assessment and starting a course of treatment.

What Are the Components of the MSE?

The MSE can be thought of as a psychiatric "review of symptoms." Assessing the five main areas listed above provides essential information for developing a differential diagnosis and a treatment plan. Expanding these five areas gives the psychological functions that are assessed and recorded in the MSE.

Sensorium & Cognitive Functioning

Level of consciousness and attentiveness
Orientation to person, place, and time
Attention
Concentration
Memory
Knowledge
Intelligence
Capacity for Abstract Thinking

Perception

Disorders of sensory input where there is no stimulus (hallucinations), where a stimulus is misperceived (illusions), or of bodily experiences

Thinking

Speech
Thought Content (*what* is said)
Thought Form (*how* something is said)
Suicidal or Homicidal Ideation
Insight & Judgment

Feeling

Affect (the objective, visible emotional state)
Mood (the subjective experience of emotion)

Behavior

Appearance
Psychomotor changes
Cooperation with the interview

How Do I Remember All That?

A mnemonic can help. The following memory aid not only lists the main areas, but does so in the order that they are usually asked about and presented.

"ABC STAMP LICKER" *

Appearance
Behavior
Cooperation

Speech
Thought — **form** and **content**
Affect — moment-to-moment variation in emotion
Mood — subjective emotional tone in the interview
Perception — in all sensory modalities

Level of consciousness
Insight & Judgment
Cognitive functioning & Sensorium
       Orientation
       Memory
       Attention & Concentration
       Reading & Writing
Knowledge base
Endings — suicidal and/or homicidal ideation
Reliability of the information

* From the book:
Psychiatric Mnemonics & Clinical Guides, 2nd Ed.
David J. Robinson, M.D.
© Rapid Psychler Press, 1998
ISBN 0-9682094-1-6

Do I Have to Conduct the MSE?

The **American Psychiatric Association (APA)** lists the MSE as one of the essential "Domains of Clinical Evaluation" (APA, 1996). It is as essential to a complete psychiatric assessment as the physical examination is in other areas of medicine. The MSE has been called a "*brain stethoscope*." (O'Neill, 1993)

All psychiatric diagnoses are made clinically in interview situations. There is no blood test, x-ray or single identifying feature for any psychiatric condition. This emphasizes the necessity of a thorough assessment, of which the MSE is an essential component. The MSE is often unpopular for two reasons:

• The questions are difficult to formulate because they are not asked in other types of interviews or in other areas of medicine, nursing, psychology, etc.
• The questions appear to be of dubious relevance to students.

Once these two difficulties are surmounted, the MSE becomes an enjoyable and interesting aspect of interviewing. To achieve this level of comfort, it helps to realize that almost half of the MSE is obtained "free" — that is through observing the patient and listening to the material from the initial parts of the interview.

"Free" Parameters	Parameters to Ask About
Level of consciousness	Orientation
Appearance	Cognitive Functioning
Behavior	Suicidal/Homicidal Thoughts
Cooperation	Knowledge Base
Reliability	Perception
Affect	Mood
Thought Form	Thought Content

How Do I Start the MSE?

The MSE begins as soon as the patient is in view. A moment of observation before the interview begins reveals important information such as: grooming, hygiene, behavior, gait, level of interest in, and interaction with, the surroundings, etc.

Other elements of the MSE are obtained as the assessment proceeds. Most interviewers begin interviews with open-ended questions and allow patients at least five minutes of relatively unstructured time to "tell their story."

Invariably, there are items that will have to be asked about specifically, which can be done in one of three ways:

1. Taking the opportunity when the chance arises in the interview. This is the most natural approach, allowing the MSE to be woven into the flow of the interview. For example, many patients will complain of poor memory and a decreased attention span, thus presenting an ideal opportunity to test cognitive functioning. The disadvantage to this method is that it can disrupt the structure of an interview. For those new to interviewing and the MSE, this approach may be better left until greater facility has been gained in redirecting patients who are giving information tangential to the assessment.

2. Taking note of key points in the history that allow a smooth transition back to these items. For example, *"You mentioned before that your vision was blurred. Did this ever cause you to see something unusual?"* This lets patients know that they have been listened to, while adhering to a more structured approach. If patients say something that introduces an important area, but at an inopportune time, say something like *"It's important for me to know about that, and we'll get back to it in a few minutes, but right now could you tell me more about . . ."* (just remember to ask about it later!)

3. Asking about the remaining areas at the end of the interview. This too has the advantage of helping preserve the structure of the interview. Additionally, the two previous approaches, while more elegant, don't always present themselves in an interview. Specific sections of the MSE can be introduced as follows:

"At this point, I'd like to ask you some questions that are separate from what we've been discussing so far, but will give me some important information about you."

or

"Right now, I'd like to ask you some questions to give me an idea about some aspects of your mental functioning."

or

"There are some other areas that I need to formally test to get an idea about your . . . (concentration, attention, etc.)."

or

"In order to be as thorough as possible, I need to ask you some questions about your mental functions and inner experiences."

These questions are only suggestions. Ask instructors or colleagues for their own patented phrases. While conducting the MSE is essential, it can be done in a variety of ways and in any order. You can draw on the experiences of others initially and then develop your own approach.

Specific questions regarding certain sections of the MSE (e.g. hallucinations and delusions) are included in their respective chapters.

Integration of the History and the MSE

Psychiatric History	MSE Component
Identifying Data & Chief Complaint	• **Appearance** • **Behavior** • **Orientation** (ask patients for their full name, if they had difficulty finding the room/clinic/hospital, etc.) • **Level of Consciousness (LOC)**
History of Present Illness (HPI) 5 — 10 minutes of relatively unstructured speech using open-ended questions and other facilitating techniques	• **Cooperation** • **Thought Form** • **Thought Content** (this format allows patients to talk about what concerns them, a valuable indicator of thought content)
Exploration of Symptoms from HPI More focused assessment with elaboration of material from the HPI using closed-ended questions to get more specific information	• **Affect** • **Mood** • **Suicidal/Homicidal Ideation** • **Elements of Cognitive Testing** (may be convenient to include certain parts at this point to gauge the severity of reported symptoms, e.g. concentration)
Direct Testing of other MSE Components For certain areas not amenable to questions earlier in the interview	• **General Knowledge** • **Perception** • **Insight & Judgment** • **Formal Cognitive Testing**

MSE Practice Points

• The **Mini-Mental State Examination (MMSE)** IS NOT the same as a complete MSE

• The MSE was originally a component of the neurological examination

• The MSE is an evaluation of the patient at the time of the interview; the findings on the MSE can and do change (invariably in front of a senior colleague); it is a record of observations made only during a particular assessment

• The MSE provides an assessment to help monitor course and prognosis; it has a high "test-retest" value and reveals important information about a patient's clinical course

• The MSE consists of a relatively standardized approach and set of inquiries, though most instructors have a rationale for doing things a certain way

• It is important to have exposure to as many styles as possible, and then assimilate this knowledge into an approach that suits you

• Different approaches can be used at different times in different ways — there is no single "right" approach

• The aim of the MSE is to have completed a thorough evaluation by the end of the interview — you are free to develop your own style

• No approach is "wrong" — you have latitude in how to conduct the MSE; you can always benefit from the ideas of others, but critically review their suggestions before automatically incorporating them into your interview style

2/ Appearance

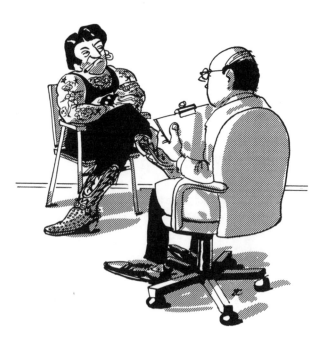

Which Aspects of Appearance Are Important?

Recording information about appearance provides a mental picture of the physical characteristics of a patient. This is done not only to obtain an accurate record, but also to convey to others as closely as possible what it was like to see the patient. Features of appearance that are important are:

- **Gender & Race** (Section I)
- **Actual & Apparent Age** (II)
- **Attire** (III)
- **Grooming & Hygiene** (IV)
- **Body Habitus** (V)
- **Physical Abnormalities** (VI)
- **Jewelry & Cosmetics** (VII)
- **Other features** (tattoos, body piercing, scars, unusual pattern of hair loss, etc.) (VIII)

How is Appearance Described?

(I) Gender, **Race** and **Age** are factual identifying features.

(II) Apparent Age is an assessment made by the interviewer based on actual age and other factors, such as the patient's hair and skin, style of clothing, and behavior. Apparent age is often recorded as:

- *Appears his or her stated age*
- *Appears younger/older than the stated age*

Many factors can contribute to an aged appearance, such as:

- Serious and/or prolonged physical illnesses
- Exposure to weather elements/homelessness
- Alcohol or other substance abuse
- Chronic and/or severe psychiatric disorders

(III) Attire describes how patients are dressed, and how they have presented themselves for the interview. Attire is a reflection of many factors: socioeconomic status, occupation, self-esteem, ability and interest in attending to convention, etc. Descriptions often include a comment on overall impression, and then the details of how patients are dressed, e.g. *"The patient was meticulously dressed in a tuxedo with a top hat and white gloves. . ."*

Due consideration must be given to the circumstances of the interview. An inpatient who awoke five minutes prior to an interview warrants a different level of expectation than would an executive attending an outpatient appointment.

It is prudent to keep in mind that medical records are legal documents. Your comments can surface again in a variety of settings, with the courtroom being one of the most common. Patients also have the right to read their medical records.

For this reason, descriptions are best made with regard to the congruity of patients' attire to the context of the interview, followed by a description of their attire. For example:

Right: *"This man is dressed as if he were prepared for the outdoors. He had on a fur hat, jacket, and striped shirt. . . "*

Wrong: *"This rube had on a très gauche, fake raccoon fur hat and a cheap-looking sweater worn over a Bert & Ernie undershirt. . ."*

Attire, when taken in context with other signs and symptoms, can provide useful information. For example:

> • During a manic episode, patients may dress flambo-
> yantly, and often show a preference for the color red

• Schizophrenia, depression, dementia and substance abuse/dependence are common causes for a declining interest in, and ability to attend to, self-care (e.g. attire, grooming, hygiene, etc.)
• Patients with personality disorders can reflect their character traits in their style and choice of clothing
• Anorectic patients often dress in loose, baggy clothing to hide their state of emaciation
• Intravenous drug users may wear long-sleeved shirts to hide needle marks ("tracks")

(IV) Grooming & Hygiene are indicators that reflect a patients level of self-care. Hair, attention to facial hair, skin condition, nails, body odor, oral hygiene, and condition of clothing are the major aspects surveyed. Common descriptions are:

• *Disheveled* (ruffled as if by a strong wind)
• *Unkempt* (poor attention to grooming)
• *Immaculately, neatly, adequately,* or *poorly groomed* are other descriptive terms used

As with attire, the level of grooming and hygiene can help to make a diagnosis and gauge the severity of the condition.

• Patients with obsessive-compulsive disorder may wash so frequently that they cause skin damage
• Delusional disorders can affect the level of grooming (e.g. not washing wards off a feared entity)
• Patients with an obsessive-compulsive or narcissistic personality disorder are often fastidiously groomed, and spend a disproportionate amount of time attending to their appearance
• Chronic, severe mental illnesses in general reduce the level at which patients maintain their self-care

(V) Body Habitus refers to the patient's build or body type. To help convey a mental image, descriptions can be made using the following terms:

> • *Ectomorphic:* thin or slight body build
> • *Mesomorphic:* muscular or sturdy build
> • *Endomorphic:* heavy or portly body build

Unusual body proportions should be noted, for example:

> • Truncal obesity and wasting of the arms and legs occurs in Cushing's Disease/Syndrome and liver diseases
> • A barrel chest which is disproportionate to the rest of the body can be caused by emphysema or chronic bronchitis

(VI) Physical Abnormalities should be noted, as well as the resulting handicap, and need for any assistive devices. In social situations, it is often polite and tactful to avoid discussing handicaps, but exploring these areas during the interview is important for completing the MSE. A sensitive line of questioning indicating your interest will help explore these areas. The following inquiries are a guide:

> • Is the missing/disfigured part a congenital or an acquired abnormality?
> • If congenital, what difficulties did this pose during development?
> • If acquired, was it through an accident? An assault? An attempt at self-harm?
> • What limitations does this currently impose?
> • How has the patient adjusted to the loss?

Exploring these areas also conveys to patients that you are willing to discuss any aspect of their lives, and creates a greater degree of openness in the interview. Physical handicaps can be significant for the following reasons:

> • The level of adjustment gives a good idea of someone's overall ability to cope with stressors and losses; the ability to adapt gives a good indication of full insight and exercising good judgment
> • Relevance to the etiology of psychiatric disorders

(VII) Jewelry and **cosmetic use** are extensions of attire and grooming, respectively. They can convey a strong and personal sense of how patients see themselves, and what they consider important. Examples of the usefulness of these observations are as follows:

> • Make-up can be bizarrely applied by patients with psychotic conditions, and lavishly by patients who are manic or have personality disorders
> • Patients with schizophrenia or schizotypal personality disorder may wear amulets and trinkets to which they have attached some mystical or highly personal significance

The study of rings is a fascinating pastime. In addition to marital status, they can indicate occupation. For example, there are school rings and engineers wear a steel or iron ring on the fifth finger of their working hand.

(VIII) Are Tattoos Significant?
The word "tattoo" is taken phonetically from a Polynesian word meaning, "to knock or strike." Tattooing has been in existence for thousands of years and extends back as far as Ancient Egypt, and possibly even further.

Tattoos are applied by the injection of permanent or indelible ink into the dermal layer of the skin. Tattoos can be applied professionally with an electric needle, or crudely manner by hand (often referred to as "jail-house"). "Tats," as they are commonly known, have achieved an unprecedented level of popularity. Many celebrities sport them. There are conventions, magazines, associations, and renowned artists, all making tattooing a culture unto itself. Tattoos have a highly personal significance. For example, they can signify membership in criminal organizations (e.g. the Japanese Mafia or Yakuza) or convictions for certain crimes. Alternatively, they can be expressions of attachment to a person or lifestyle (e.g. sexual orientation or sexual practices).

Isn't It Judgmental to Make Inferences About A Patient's Appearance?

Appearance is too important a feature to not include when gathering information during the MSE. While inferences can be drawn and hypotheses made regarding certain features, further information is required for confirmation.

Diagnosis and treatment require more than appearance alone. People adapt their grooming style to express themselves by wearing certain clothing, jewelry, and cosmetics. In interview situations, clinicians strive to interpret more than fashion statements. A wealth of information is available to experienced observers.

To illustrate this, consider the famous Victorian detective Sherlock Holmes. In the short-story called *The Yellow Face*, he examines a pipe and tells Watson "the owner is obviously a muscular man, left-handed, with an excellent set of teeth, careless in his habits, and with no need to practice economy."

How Holmes arrives at these conclusions makes perfect sense once he reveals both his observations and their significance.

3/ Behavior

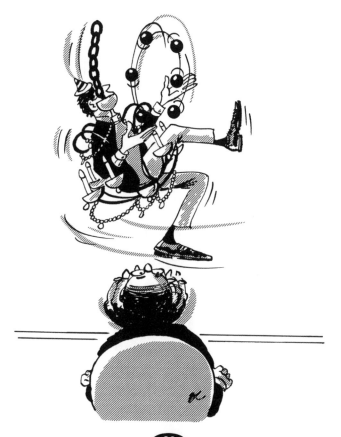

Which Aspects of Behavior Are Important?

Behavior refers to activity during the interview, and is one of the cardinal means of determining mental illness. It provides outwardly observable manifestations of psychiatric conditions. Patients may be delusional, suicidal or plagued by hallucinations, but these are internal experiences to which a clinician has no direct access. Behavior reveals information about other parameters of the MSE, such as mood, cooperation & reliability, thought content, etc. As with appearance, the assessment of behavior begins the instant patients are first seen, which may be the only opportunity to observe certain actions (e.g. tics, compulsions). The major aspects of behavior are:

General Observations
- **Agitation** (Section I)
- **Hyperactivity** (II)
- **Psychomotor Retardation** (III)

Observation of Specific Movements
- **Akathisia** (Section IV)
- **Automatisms** (V)
- **Catatonia** (VI)
- **Choreoathetoid Movements** (VII)
- **Compulsions** (VIII)
- **Dystonias** (IXa) & **Extrapyramidal Symptoms** (IXb)
- **Tardive Dyskinesia** (X)
- **Tics** (XI)
- **Tremors** (XII)
- **Negative Symptoms** (XIII)

Observation of behavior is the critical element in descriptive psychopathology. **Phenomenology**, the study of observed events without inferring a cause, was the initial basis for classifying mental disorders.

How Do I Describe the General Aspects of Activity?

Activity level is a global description of patients' physical movements. Individual factors assessed are:

- Posture
- Range and frequency of spontaneous movements
- Cooperation and ability to carry out requested tasks

Activity level is generally recorded as:

- *Increased* (also referred to as agitated)
- *Decreased* or *slowed* (hypokinesis, bradykinesia)
- *Within normal limits* (WNL)

Even in cases where there are no obvious behavioral abnormalities, a brief description provides a visual image of what it was like to be in the interview. For example, *"Mr. Y.K.K. sat comfortably in the room with his arms folded across his chest and absent mindedly fiddled with the zipper on his jacket . . ."*

It is helpful to classify movements in three ways:

- **Conscious voluntary movements** — such as getting up to clean the dust off the lamp shade
- **Unconscious voluntary movements** — such as adjusting eyeglasses or clearing the throat; *Habits & Mannerisms* fall into this category
- **Involuntary movements** — such as tremors or dystonias; these are usually found to be neurological abnormalities

The MSE records only the behavior, not the patients' internal experiences (i.e. patients who adjust their glasses may have a motor tic, however, only the action itself is recorded).

(I) Agitation is used to describe physical restlessness, usually with a heightened sense of tension and level of arousal. Common signs are:

- Hand wringing, finger tapping or fidgeting
- Frequent shifts in posture or position
- Foot tapping or rhythmic leg movements
- Frequent shifts in the focus of attention

Agitation can also be used to describe an emotional state or **affect**, in that patients can both feel and appear agitated. **Psychomotor** refers to movements that are psychically determined, as opposed to those caused by external sources. For example, a high intake of caffeine can cause people to feel restless and agitated. This distinction is important because there are many causes for agitation (see list below). In recognition of this, the DSM-IV specifies **psychomotor agitation** in the diagnostic criteria for mania, hypomania, and depression. Agitation is seen in the following conditions:

- Substance ingestion/withdrawal
- General medical conditions such as hyperthyroidism, hypoparathyroidism, dementia, and delirium
- Psychiatric conditions such as schizophrenia, depression, mania/hypomania, any of the anxiety disorders, and Cluster A & C personality disorders

Cluster A — Paranoid, Schizoid, Schizotypal
Cluster B — Histrionic, Borderline, Antisocial, Narcissistic
Cluster C — Obsessive-Compulsive, Dependent, Avoidant

- Agitated depression: patients may experience a **mixed state** of manic and depressive symptoms; this is very unpleasant to endure and more highly correlated with completed suicide than are other bipolar mood states.

(II) Hyperactivity refers to an increased level of physical energy. It is distinguished from agitation by the absence of inner tension, and by the fact that the extra energy is usually goal-directed. Patients often speak quickly and at length, and may become unusually assertive or even aggressive. This is a common observation among patients suffering from:

- Mania or hypomania
- Attention-Deficit/Hyperactivity Disorder (ADHD)
- Obsessive-Compulsive personalities

An increased level of activity can also be seen in the following conditions:

- Catatonic excitement
- Seizure disorders, particularly during an interictal period
- Head injuries or delirium

Psychomotor retardation refers to slowness of voluntary and involuntary movements. Other terms used to describe retardation are **hypokinesia** or **bradykinesia** and, in extreme cases, the virtual absence of movement is called **akinesia**. The term retardation applies to the initiation, execution, and completion of movement. It excludes those who may have trouble starting tasks due to indecisiveness, but who are capable of completing them readily (such as obsessive-compulsive personalities) and those who start tasks readily but can't complete them (such as patients with dementia).

Often accompanying the slowed movements are changes in voice and **prosody of speech** (the natural emotional tone or inflection of speech). Most people move spontaneously when speaking, often gesturing with their hands to facilitate speech or to accentuate what they are saying. Other typical movements include adjusting eyeglasses, scratching, shifting posture, crossing and uncrossing legs, folding and unfolding arms, etc. Keeping track of a patient's repertoire of spontaneous movements is valuable in assessments. Make a point of asking about unusual or repetitive actions, or the absence of typical movements. Descriptions of behavior must also be prefaced by an indication of the level of consciousness. You would not be surprised to hear that obtunded or comatose patients demonstrated severely diminished body movements (akinesia in these cases), but you'd probably like to hear about their level of consciousness first.

In general, mental processes are slowed along with movements, with patients reporting that they are unable to think as fast as usual. Such reports must be distinguished from **mental retardation** (sub-average mental functioning prior to age 18). The distinction is that patients who are mentally retarded have permanent learning disabilities. Patients with dementia achieved a normal level of intelligence, and then acquired an illness causing them to lose their mental faculties. Depression can affect cognitive functioning so severely that the person appears to be demented. This is called **pseudodementia** or, more recently, the **dementia syndrome of depression**. While this latter term more accurately reflects the pathology of the process, pseudodementia is seen in other conditions and is still widely used as a descriptive term. Causes for decreased or diminished movements are:

> • Depression, which is the most common psychiatric cause; in past diagnostic nomenclature, there was a subtype of depression called *retarded depression*
> • Schizophrenia and in particular, the presence of **negative symptoms**
> • Medication side-effects, especially to antipsychotics
> • Catatonia
> • Dementia, of any cause
> • General medical conditions

Specific Movement Abnormalities

(IV) Akathisia is a state of inner drivenness to keep in motion. It occurs as a side-effect of antipsychotic medication. Patients often seem ill at ease, move their legs rhythmically or have to get up and walk around the room. Akathisia cannot be differentiated from other states of agitation by observation alone — it is a subjective experience. It is called *neuroleptic-induced* when it is caused by antipsychotic medications. The usual manifestations are rocking, fidgeting, pacing or generally feeling compelled to keep moving. Akathisia can be quite uncomfortable. Suicides and assaults have been reported because it was not detected or adequately treated. It is often caused by starting or increasing the dosage of antipsychotic medication, or by decreasing or stopping agents which reduce the symptoms. Voluntary suppression of akathisia-driven movements only increases the sense of discomfort.

(V) Automatisms are "automatic" involuntary movements that can range from relatively simple to complex behaviors. They occur most commonly in epileptic seizures of the partial complex or absence type. Automatisms may be the only outward manifestations of a seizure disorder. They are also seen in head injuries, substance ingestion, catatonia, and dissociative and fugue states. By definition, automatisms occur during an altered state of consciousness. During automatisms, actions can range from purposeful to disorganized, and may or may not be appropriate for the situation or the person displaying them. Patients may be partially aware of their surroundings. They may continue with their actions, but do not seem "quite right" at the time, and are amnestic for the episode. Typical automatisms are:

- Lip-smacking or uttering words
- Fumbling with clothing
- Eye blinking or staring with an unwavering stare

(VI) Catatonia is a term applied to a diverse number of postural and movement disturbances. The movement disorders can include both increased and decreased levels of activity. The term catatonia was developed by Kahlbaum, and was initially a diagnostic entity on its own. If Kahlbaum had been a dog person, he would have called it dogatonia. Catatonia is also found in:

- Periodic catatonia, a rare variant involving an alteration of thyroid function and nitrogen balance
- Neurologic illnesses
- Syphilis and viral encephalopathies
- Head trauma, arteriovenous malformations, etc.
- Toxic states and metabolic abnormalities

A mnemonic for the DSM-IV criteria for catatonia is:

"WRENCHES"

Weird (peculiar) movements
Rigidity
Echopraxia — copying someone's body movements
Negativism — automatic opposition to all requests
Catalepsy — waxy flexibility
High level of motor activity
Echolalia — repeating the words of others
Stupor — immobility

(VII) Choreoathetoid movements are seen in various neurologic and psychiatric disorders. This is an amalgamation of two types of movement disorders, choreiform and athetoid.

Choreiform movements are involuntary and appear as irregular, jerky, spasmodic, and quasi-purposeful; they are irregularly timed and generally not repeated; these movements most often affect the face and arms. An example of a choreiform movement is someone whose hand shoots up towards his face, and who incorporates this into an adjustment of his hair.

Athetoid movements are slow, writhing (snake-like), twisting, and have the appearance of following a pattern. Any muscle group can be affected. An athetoid movement might look like someone practicing Tai Chi, or using a their hand to imitate an airplane climbing and diving.

Ballismus is a larger-amplitude, faster, and more violent motion (it has the same word root as ballistics). It usually occurs on one side of the body (hemiballismus) and resembles speeded-up athetoid movements (like a punch into the air). The most common causes for these movements are:

- Huntington's Chorea
- Sydenham's Chorea (rheumatic fever)
- Wilson's Disease (hepatolenticular degeneration)
- Multiple Sclerosis
- Tourette's Disorder

Causes of particular interest in psychiatry are:

- Use of antiparkinsonian (dopaminergic) agents
- Use of stimulants (e.g. for ADHD)
- Use of anticonvulsants (e.g. phenytoin)
- Lithium toxicity
- Tardive Dyskinesia

(VIII) Compulsions are defined in the DSM-IV as:
(1) Repetitive behaviors or mental acts that the person feels driven to perform in response to an obsession, or according to rules that must be applied rigidly.
(2) Behaviors or mental acts aimed at preventing or reducing distress or preventing some dreaded event or situation; how-

ever, these behaviors or mental acts are either not connected in a realistic way with what they are designed to neutralize or prevent, or are clearly excessive.

Two points require emphasis with this definition:

1. Compulsions can be entirely mental experiences, such as prayers or sayings, though the majority are actions.
2. The "rules that must be applied rigidly" are self-imposed and not due to involvement with an organization with a strict code of conduct (e.g. mom, the military, boarding schools).

Compulsions are:

> • Unwanted, and egodystonic (insight is preserved)
> • Purposeful or semi-purposeful actions that are performed to decrease anxiety
> • Performed consciously
> • Stereotyped (repeated over and over)
> • Ritualistic (performed the same way each time)
> • Usually linked to obsessions; e.g. obsessions about dirt cause compulsions to clean things, etc.

Compulsions can occur individually, but are usually preceded by obsessions, defined as recurrent thoughts, images or impulses that are:

> • Recurrent, and recognized as unreasonable
> • Not simply excessive concerns about realistic problems
> • Recognized as a product of the person's mind, as opposed to thoughts being inserted from elsewhere

A patient's current compulsions may or may not be evident in interview situations. Some patients can endure the anxiety that stems from suppressing compulsions for the duration of the time spent being observed. If compulsions are reported but not seen, they should be listed in the case presentation in the present or past psychiatric illness section, but not in the MSE. The most common compulsions are:

- Excessive or ritualized grooming (hand washing, showering, brushing teeth, etc.)
- Excessive cleaning of objects
- Repetition (e.g. dressing in a certain order)
- Checking (doors to see if locked)
- Counting, touching & measuring
- Ordering or arranging (usually in some logical sequence, e.g. size, alphabetical order, for symmetry and precision)
- Hoarding and collecting

The following questions can help screen for compulsions:

- *Are there actions that you perform repetitively?*
- *Do you spend time doing something over and over?*
- *Do you, for example, clean, check, count or arrange things on a repetitive basis?*

(IXa) Dystonia is an involuntary increase in muscle tone, and a subtype of **extrapyramidal side effect**. Dystonias are manifested as sustained torsions or contractions of muscles (usually muscle groups) that give patients a contorted appearance. They generally occur in three circumstances:

- As a reaction to antipsychotic medications
- As a consequence of chronic schizophrenia
- As the consequence of a neurologic condition

Acute dystonias usually occur within the first five days of neuroleptic administration. Young males, and patients who receive high potency neuroleptics (e.g. haloperidol), are at higher risk for these reactions. Some clinicians advocate that antiparkinsonian agents be used prophylactically to prevent such reactions in higher-risk groups. Common dystonias are:

- **Oculogyric crisis** or **spasm** — fixed upward gaze, or eye muscles forced into a dysconjugate gaze
- **Torticollis** or **wry neck** — a spasmodic contraction of neck muscles causing the head to rotate and the chin to point to the side opposite the spasm
- **Opisthotonos** — a spasm in the neck and back that causes an arching forward; in severe cases, recumbent patients have only their heels and the backs of their heads touching the floor
- **Laryngospasm** — a dystonia of the muscles controlling the tongue and throat; it can lead to difficulty speaking, swallowing, and breathing

Dystonias are very uncomfortable and frightening for patients. The presence of a dystonic reaction requires immediate intervention. Prolonged reactions such as those listed above are a major reason that patients do not comply with their medications. Untreated, these reactions can last at least an hour. Fortunately, dystonias can usually be treated effectively and quickly with antiparkinsonian medications.

Most acute dystonias seen in current practice are due to antipsychotic medication. However, dystonias have been documented in patients with schizophrenia who have never been exposed to neuroleptic medication. Not only have dystonic reactions been recorded, but a whole range of motor disorders have been seen, including abnormalities in:

- Posture, tone and gait
- Eye movements and blinking
- Facial, head, trunk, and limb movements
- Speech production

Dystonias can also be **tardive** as opposed to acute. Next to **torticollis**, the most common is **blepharospasm** (involuntary closure of both eyes), though this often spreads to muscles controlling head movements and chewing. Dystonia itself is a neurologic condition. It is differentiated from other motor disorders by the presence of repetitive, patterned, and sustained movements when due to neurologic causes.

(IXb) Other Extrapyramidal Symptoms (EPS)

The pyramidal tracts are made up of axons that originate in the posterior frontal and anterior parietal lobes. Ninety percent of the fibers pass through the pyramid of the medulla and form a tract found laterally in the spinal cord. The group of nuclei known as the **basal ganglia** make up the major component of the extrapyramidal system. The following is a list of extrapyramidal reactions (in their usual order of occurrence after neuroleptic administration):

- Dystonic reactions (hours to days)
- Akathisia (hours to weeks)
- Akinesia or Bradykinesia (days to weeks)
- Rigidity (days to weeks)
- Tremors (weeks to months)
- Pisa and Rabbit Syndrome (months to years)

Parkinsonism refers to the symptoms, but not the presence of Parkinson's Disease (defined as an idiopathic depletion of dopaminergic neurons in the basal ganglia occurring in a sporadic and familial form). The causes of parkinsonism that are of most relevance to psychiatry are:

1. Medication-induced dopamine blockade — neuroleptics are dopamine receptor blockers (the antidepressant amoxapine and several antiemetics — prochlorperazine, metoclopramide, promethazine, trimethobenzamide, thiethylperazine, trifluopromazine also have this action).

2. Medication-induced dopamine depletion, which occurs with reserpine and tetrabenazine.

3. Lithium, disulfiram, methyldopa, and some of the calcium channel blockers.

4. Toxins such as carbon monoxide, cyanide and methanol.

Other extrapyramidal symptoms (EPS) are:

> • **Pisa Syndrome**, so named because patients' posture bears a resemblance to the Leaning Tower of Pisa. It is a **tardive dystonia** that causes a torsion spasm of the torso muscles.
>
> • **Rabbit Syndrome**, a quick, alternating perioral movement that resembles the chewing action of a rabbit's mouth, often with a smacking of the lips. This is more rapid and regular than the oro-facial-bucco-lingual movements seen in **tardive dyskinesia.**

(X) Tardive Dyskinesia (TD) is an involuntary movement disorder associated with chronic neuroleptic use. *Tardive* refers to the delayed onset, which occurs from months to years after starting medication. *Dyskinesia* is a distortion of voluntary movement. This condition is composed of **choreoathetoid** movements, but is considered separately due to its importance in psychiatry. TD occurs in three areas of the body:

Facial & oral movements (present in 75% of those affected)
> • Facial expressions — frowning, grimacing
> • Lips and mouth — puckering, lip smacking
> • Jaw — chewing, teeth grinding
> • Tongue — tremor, protrusion, rolling

Extremities (present in 50% of those affected)
> • Choreoathetoid movements in the limbs
> • Tremors or rhythmic movements may be present
> • Range from rapid, purposeless and spontaneous to slow and complex motions

Trunk (present in 25% of those affected)
> • Twisting, rocking or gyrating of the back, neck, shoulders or pelvis

In the early stages of development, TD can easily be missed. It is often not reported by patients, but by those around them who are aware of the repetitive movements (often smacking or chewing). It can easily be passed off as gum or tobacco chewing or as ill-fitting dentures.

The movements of TD are more pronounced during stressful periods and with use of non-affected body parts. Lessening of the movements is seen during periods of relaxation, use of the affected parts, and voluntary suppression. TD is typically absent during sleep. An increase in neuroleptic dosage temporarily improves the symptoms, whereas the use of an **anticholinergic agent (ACA)** can worsen some forms of TD.

In severe cases, TD can also cause irregularities in speaking, breathing, and swallowing. Swallowing air (**aerophagia**) can lead to chronic belching or grunting. Limb involvement can leave patients incapacitated. The risk factors that increase the likelihood of TD are:

> • Advancing age and female gender
> • Duration of neuroleptic administration
> • Increasing neuroleptic dosage
> • Presence of a non-psychotic disorder
> • Drug holidays (these are not "summer trips," but planned discontinuations of medication)

A research instrument was designed to assess the presence of TD. It is called the **Abnormal Involuntary Movement Scale (AIMS)**. The AIMS involves both observation and asking the patient to perform actions that assist the detection of TD. This condition is not rare and, therefore, is worth taking the time to detect. Up to 5% of younger patients who take neuroleptics for one year have at least one finding. This increases to 30% in elderly patients. TD has been reported in schizophrenic patients who have never taken neuroleptic medication. It has been proposed to be a late complication of schizophrenia that has been spuriously associated with neuroleptic administration. Nevertheless, there have been successful lawsuits brought forward because of a lack of **informed consent**.

(XI) Tics are involuntary, sudden, rapid, recurrent, non-rhythmic, stereotyped, irresistible movements or vocalizations. Tics generally mimic all or part of a normal movement, and may be seen as "purposeful" in this regard. They can range from simple to complex, though their duration is often only about one second. Most patients with tics have a unique "repertoire" that varies in type, location, degree, and frequency. Tics often occur in paroxysmal bouts.

Patients can voluntarily suppress tics during interviews, however this becomes increasingly difficult, and is associated with escalating discomfort. Prior to a tic occurring, patients may experience premonitory urges or sensations. As with compulsions, a feeling of relief comes with expression of the tic. Stress, fatigue, new situations or even boredom can exacerbate tics. Other illnesses, concentration on other matters, relaxation, alcohol, and orgasm can diminish tics. Like other movement disorders, tics are virtually absent during sleep. Examples of simple motor tics are:

- Blinking or **blepharospasm**
- Facial twitches, grimaces, head jerking
- Shrugging or rotation of the shoulders
- Grinding teeth (**bruxism**)

Examples of complex motor tics are:
- Head shaking
- Jumping or kicking
- Hitting or biting oneself
- Touching or smelling objects

Examples of simple vocal tics are:
- Coughing, humming
- Grunting, gurgling
- Throat clearing, clicking or clacking
- Sneezing, sniffing, snorting or snuffling

Examples of complex vocal tics are:
- Utterances of inappropriate syllables or words
- **Copralalia** (saying or shouting obscenities)
- **Palilalia** (repeating one's own phrases)

Tics occur in a wide variety of conditions:
- Physiologic tics — mannerisms or gestures
- Primary tic disorders (e.g. Tourette's Disorder)
- Chromosomal abnormalities — Down's Syndrome
- Medications — e.g. stimulants used for the treatment of ADHD
- Head trauma
- Mental Retardation
- Neurologic conditions — e.g. Huntington's Disease, Sydenham's Chorea, Wilson's Disease
- Infections — e.g. encephalitis
- Schizophrenia
- Gasoline or carbon monoxide poisoning

(XII) Tremors are involuntary movements consisting of regular, rhythmic oscillations of some part of the body. They are usually seen in the hands, arms, head, neck, lips, mouth or tongue, but can also occur in the legs, voice or trunk.

The causes of tremors which are most relevant to psychiatry are as follows:

> • Stress-induced — situational anxiety, anxiety disorders (e.g. panic disorder), strong emotions, fatigue, and hypothermia
> • Psychotropic medication-induced — lithium, valproate, neuroleptics, tricyclic antidepressants (TCAs), selective serotonin reuptake inhibitors (SSRIs)
> • Familial or physiologic tremors
> • Neurologic or endocrine

(XIII) Negative Symptoms
Part of developing skills as an interviewer is to not only pay attention to what is being said or done, but also to what is *not* being said or done. For example, patients who talk about their families while omitting certain members (like a parent) often betray the presence of a conflict with that person. Similarly, there are certain behaviors that are remarkable for their absence instead of presence.

Many clinicians divide the signs and symptoms of schizophrenia into **positive** and **negative symptoms**, also referred to as **Type I** and **Type II** schizophrenia, respectively. One way to conceptualize this distinction is that positive symptoms are "added" to the picture while negative ones are deficits in the clinical presentation. **Positive symptoms** are: **hallucinations**, **delusions**, **formal thought disorders** and **bizarre** or **disorganized behavior**. A mnemonic for negative symptoms is:

"NEGATIVE TRACK"

> **N**egligible response to conventional antipsychotics
> **E**ye contact is decreased
> **G**rooming & hygiene decline

Affective responses become flat
Thought blocking
Inattentiveness
Volition diminished
Expressive gestures decrease

Time — increases the number of negative symptoms
Recreational interests/Relationships diminish
A's — see below for the 5 A's
Content of speech diminishes (poverty of thought)
Knowledge — cognitive deficits increase

• When Kraepelin and Bleuler first described schizophrenia, they made distinctions between fundamental (positive) and accessory (negative) symptoms. By the way, Bleuler suggested the term schizophrenia in 1911 to refer to a splitting of the mind. Prior to this, Kraepelin called it **dementia praecox**.

• Negative symptoms are not usually treated effectively by traditional antipsychotic medications (positive symptoms respond more favorably). Newer antipsychotics (risperidone, clozapine, quetiapine, olanzapine) appear to treat negative symptoms much more effectively. Dr. Nancy Andreason developed standardized scales to assess the presence of positive and negative symptoms. The scale for positive symptoms is called the **SAPS (Scale for the Assessment of Positive Symptoms)**. The other is the **SANS (Scale for the Assessment of Negative Symptoms)**. The major headings in this scale are in the following mnemonic:

a**P**athy
a**L**ogia
  Affective flattening
a**N**hedonia
a**T**tentional deficits

'**PLANT**' mnemonic for the five A's from the *Scale for the Assessment of Negative Symptoms* provided by:

Dr. David Wagner, Indiana University

4/ Cooperation & Reliability

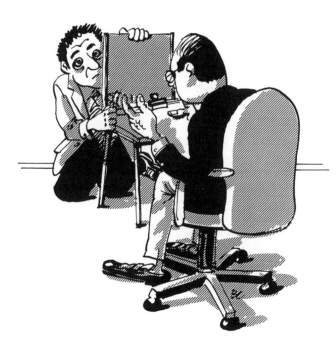

What Factors Determine Cooperation & Reliability?

Cooperation from patients is required so that the information they provide is useful in forming a diagnostic impression. Some patients can't or won't share information. The degree of co-operation offered by patients needs to be made clear early in the presentation of the MSE, as it colors the rest of the information obtained. In a sense, cooperation refers to the *quantity* of information given. Cooperation is possibly best gauged by the responses patients give to open-ended questions, which allows them a relatively unstructured opportunity to say what is on their minds. Most patients share information freely and participate readily in the interview.

Of course, a cornucopia of information is not useful unless it is accurate. In a similar vein, reliability refers to the *quality* of data obtained in the interview. The following parameters provide an assessment of cooperation and reliability:

- **Eye Contact** (Section I)
- **Attitude/Demeanor** (II)
- **Attentiveness to the Interview** (III)
- **Level of Consciousness** (IV)
- **Affect** (V)
- **Secondary Gain** (VI)

How Do I Describe the Various Aspects of Cooperation & Reliability?

(I) Eye Contact is a universal indicator that someone is interested. Continued eye contact indicates cooperativeness. Patients may avert their gaze momentarily to think about something. Sustained aversion of gaze can indicate that the patient has encountered an area of difficulty. Eye contact is described as *continuous, good, intermittent, fleeting, or absent*.

(II) Attitude/Demeanor towards the interview and interviewer is another important aspect of cooperation. Patients may have biases from previous contact with mental health professionals. This usually becomes obvious early in the interview, and can pose a significant obstacle to obtaining information. Such a bias is most commonly seen with patients who:

- Have personality disorders (typically borderline or antisocial)
- Are under duress to attend the interview
- Suffer from chronic conditions that have resulted in numerous contacts with different caregivers
- Have an agenda (**secondary gain**) to carry out
- Are cognitively impaired due to organic processes or substance ingestion/withdrawal

Demeanor can be described as being *cooperative* or *uncooperative*. Cooperative patients can be further described as:

- *Obsequious/Solicitous/Effusive*
- *Seductive/Flattering/Charming*
- *Over-inclusive/Eager to please*
- *Entitled/Controlling*

The manner in which patients are uncooperative requires elaboration. For example:

- *Hostile/Defensive*
- *Suspicious/Guarded*
- *Antagonistic/Critical*
- *Childish/Regressed*
- *Sullen/Withdrawn*

To illustrate your description, include a quote or observation from the interview.

(III) Attentiveness to the Interview impacts on the degree of cooperation and reliability. Patients can be distracted by external (noise) or internal stimuli (hallucinations) while speaking. Further, they may preferentially attend to these events and not see the point of answering your questions. Interest can diminish in an interview for any of a number of reasons:

- Borderline or antisocial personalities often become bored in interview situations
- Patients experiencing a manic or hypomanic episode may be so distractible that they cannot attend to the questions being asked of them
- Delirious patients can drift in and out of lucidity
- Obsessive-Compulsive Disorder can cause patients to succumb to the intrusive thoughts or the irresistible urge to reduce their state of anxiety; they may engage in a number of ritualized behaviors
- Patients who are psychotic may experience hallucinations or incorporate interview material into delusions, which then reduces their ability to attend to questions

This is recorded in the MSE as patients being attentive/inattentive. A further description is given for diminished attention span. Reasons might include:

- Being preoccupied
- A reduced or fluctuating level of consciousness
- Being distracted by activity in the interview
- Sudden shifts in affect or mood state

(IV) Level of Consciousness (LOC) refers to the degree of alertness or level of arousal. In typical interview situations, patients are alert, attentive to their surroundings and responsive to questions. This can be recorded in the MSE as *"the patient was fully alert and attentive to the interview."*

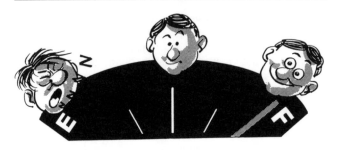

Aberrations in the level of arousal are important to include early in the recording or reporting of the MSE. The reader or listener needs to be aware of this at the outset, because an altered level of consciousness affects the quality of the information that follows. A diminished LOC immediately calls into question the possibility of an organic condition and warrants urgent investigation.

(VI) Affect is defined as:

> • The observable quality of an emotional state
> • The moment-to-moment variability of visible emotions based on what is occurring in the interview (external events) or feelings (internal events)
> • The range of reactions to questions that would usually be considered of emotional significance

A financial analogy is as follows: affect is the minute-to-minute variation in the worth of a company stock, mood is the general trend over a longer time period. Another analogy is that affect is like weather, and mood is like climate.

Affect is reported in a separate chapter along with mood. In situations where intense affect interferes with obtaining information, describing it in the *Cooperation & Reliability* section helps put subsequent information into perspective.

(VI) Secondary gain refers to an actual or external advantage that patients gain from being ill. Common examples include:

- Being relieved of occupational responsibilities
- Obtaining prescription medication
- Avoiding military service
- Leverage in personal relationships
- Postponing exams
- Transfer out of prison or jail
- Shelter and/or food
- Financial gain

In psychoanalytic theory, a symptom functions to decrease intrapsychic conflict and distress, which is considered the **primary gain**. **Tertiary gain** is the advantage others receive from the patient's illness (e.g. disability income supporting a family).

What Is the Relevance of "Gain" to the MSE?

Malingering is the conscious production of physical or psychiatric symptoms for secondary gain. Any mental disorder can be mimicked by organic conditions, or by someone skilled in describing psychiatric symptoms. There is no way of objectively assessing auditory hallucinations, paranoia, flashbacks or other internal experiences. No laboratory test or other investigation can verify the symptoms reported by patients. For this reason, mental illnesses are often favored by malingerers.

Factitious Disorder is the deliberate production of symptoms (physical or psychological) in the apparent absence of secondary gain. Symptoms are produced so that patients can assume "the sick role." The motivation is thought to be for **primary gain**; however, there may be secondary gain that is not immediately obvious.

5/ Speech

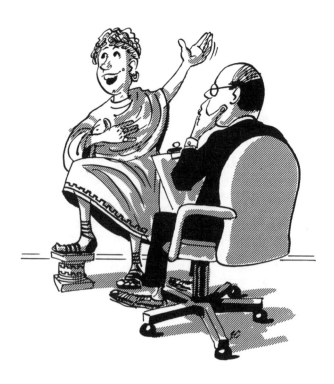

Which Aspects of Speech Are Important?

Speech

Language   **Thought Process**

Speech refers to verbal expression, which consists of utterances, words, phrases, and sentences.

Language refers to the communication of comprehensible ideas. Not all speech is language (e.g. vocal tics, campaign promises). Language can be conveyed by means other than speech — posture, gestures, expressions, actions, and sign language all transmit clear meaning without requiring verbal expression. Language consists of ideas (usually expressed as words) that convey meaning (**semantics**), and are properly produced (**articulation**).

Thought process refers to the way ideas are produced and organized. Thought is inferred from speech and language (including writing or signing) because it cannot be assessed directly.

Thought and language have a large interplay but describe different processes. Language is the principal means by which thought process is expressed. Animals and preverbal humans readily demonstrate that thought occurs without the ability to express syntactical language.

While humans are anatomically capable of speech, language is an acquired ability. Understandable sounds and words are uttered by eighteen months while phrases are spoken between two and three years of age.

How Are Speech Centers Organized in the CNS?

The brain is lateralized, with the areas responsible for speech being found in the dominant cerebral hemisphere. Lateralization is related to hand dominance:

• Right-handers make up 90% of the population and almost all have their speech centers on the left side of the brain
• About two-thirds of left-handers have a dominant left cerebral hemisphere, while the remainder have right-sided or bilateral dominance
• Gauging dominance by observing the writing hand is about 85% accurate, while observing footedness (e.g. in kicking a ball) is about 98% accurate
• Handedness is a hereditary trait, but the hand used for writing can be switched if necessary (e.g. a broken hand)

While the dominant hemisphere (usually left) controls most of the functions of speech, the right hemisphere provides an integrative function. In order to "get the whole picture," or see "the forest and the trees," the nondominant hemisphere must be functioning. Other nondominant functions include the inflection, rhythm, and emotional components of language. Interestingly, second and later languages and obscenities are not controlled by the dominant hemisphere. Damage to the corpus callosum (the neurons connecting the hemispheres of the brain) can result in a number of language abnormalities.

The following cranial nerves (CN) are required for the comprehension and production of speech:

• CN 5 — control of articulation via jaw muscles
• CN 7 — control of articulation via facial muscles
• CN 8 — (cochlear part) for auditory information
• CN 9, 10, 11 & 12 — control the soft palate, pharynx, larynx, and tongue to implement speech

Assessing speech abnormalities begins with the following:

1. *Is the patient's speech abnormal?*
2. *In what way is it abnormal?*
3. *Was the patient's speech ever normal?*
       If not, consider one of the conditions affecting the
       acquisition of normal language skills (listed below)
4. *Is anything else abnormal in addition to speech?*
   - Reading
   - Comprehension
   - Copying
   - Response to directions
   - Writing/Drawing
   - Repetition
   - Naming

Given that speech is encoded thought, the chance to hear patients speak gives us valuable clues about their mental functioning. It is not an unusual experience to have a patient present for an interview who is shabbily dressed and acting in an eccentric manner. While you are busy (prematurely) considering some heavy-duty diagnosis, you are taken aback by the person's intelligence and eloquent speech.

Which Conditions Affect the Acquisition of Normal Language Skills?

   - Mental Retardation
   - Autism
   - Pervasive Developmental Disorders
       (e.g Rett's Disorder, Heller's Syndrome
       Asperger's Disorder)

Distinguishing Medical From Psychiatric Causes of Speech Disturbance

Distinguishing between aphasias and disorders of thought process can be difficult because they both affect verbal expression. In the case of severe psychiatric disturbances, it may not be possible in one interview to make the distinction. A classic example is the differentiating speech abnormalities in psychosis from true aphasia. The following is a list of potential distinguishing features:

Parameter	Medical	Psychiatric
• Greater severity	+	-
• Continuous duration	+	-
• Abrupt onset	+	-
• Older age of onset	+	-
• Related language symptoms	+	-
• Word finding difficulties	+	-
• Awareness of difficulty (partial)	+	-
• Loss of repetition, naming and comprehension abilities	+	-

What Are the Specific Aphasias?

Because of the potential difficulties in distinguishing primary language disorders from psychiatric conditions, the aphasias will be summarized here. The reason that it is vital to make this distinction is that aphasias almost always involve an injury to the dominant cerebral hemisphere, which requires urgent intervention. Psychiatric conditions are less medically urgent and involve significantly different forms of treatment.

Aphasias are usually classified as **fluent** or **nonfluent**. Further distinction is made using three tests:
• **Comprehension** — tested by the ability to follow simple, and later, complex requests
• **Repetition** — tested with simple and complex phrases
• **Naming** — tested with common and uncommon objects

An alternate system classification aphasias as either **receptive** or **expressive** based on the ability to understand and speak, respectively. This system poses difficulties for non-neurologists because there are frequently both receptive and expressive deficits present when interviewing aphasic patients.

Paraphasias (paraphasic errors) are the substitution of a letter or word for the intended word. There are four types:

- Related (approximative) — *light* is used instead of *lamp*
- Unrelated (semantic) — *caboose* is used instead of *lamp*
- Literal (phonemic) — *lump* is used instead of *lamp*
- Neologistic (jargon) — *piloknarf* is used instead of *lamp*

Nonfluent Aphasias
- Broca's
- Transcortical Motor
- Global

Fluent Aphasias
- Wernicke's
- Transcortical Sensory
- Conduction
- Anomic

What Other Qualities of Speech Are There?

(I) Accent & Dialect are terms used interchangeably to describe regional or cultural differences in pronunciation. Accent can be used to refer to the speech of patients who are not native English speakers (e.g. a French, Swedish or Spanish accent). Dialect can be used to describe regional variations in those who are native anglophones.

There are five major dialects in the U.S. — New York, New England, Southern, Appalachian and Western. In Canada, those from the Atlantic Provinces have a distinct style of speech, while the rest of the country has a "middle American" accent. In the U.K., the skill in distinguishing dialect is finely honed. Britons can almost make an educated guess as to the side of the street someone lived on while growing up.

(II) Amount of speech varies widely in interview situations. Mental health professionals spend years learning how to obtain and organize salient information. Patients are given considerable leeway for what constitutes a "normal" amount of speech (recorded as *responsive, spontaneous, well-spoken,* or *fluent*). Anxious patients provide extraneous detail through their desire to be helpful. Other patients feel inhibited, provide sparse answers, and offer little information spontaneously. The amount of speech can be increased in:

- Mania (see **pressure of speech** below)
- Anxiety Disorders
- Personality Disorders
- Fluent aphasias

Terms used to describe an increased amount of speech are: *verbose, loquacious, talkative, copious, logorrhea, vociferous, overabundant,* or *expansive.* The amount of speech can be decreased in:

- Depression
- Schizophrenia (particularly as a negative symptom)
- Avoidant, dependent, and schizoid personalities
- Dementia (especially the early stages) or delirium

Terms used to describe a decreased amount of speech are: *paucity of speech, impoverished, laconic, taciturn, single word answers,* and *minimally responsive.*

At one extreme, **pressure of speech** describes patients who are driven to keep talking, and have an increased rate and amount of speech. A key feature of pressured speech is that it is not usually interruptible. The other extreme involves the absence of speech, which is called **mutism**. This is found in neurologic conditions and extreme forms of psychiatric illnesses (particularly depression and schizophrenia).

(III) Articulation refers to the clarity with which words are spoken. This is not a description of word finding ability or eloquence of speech. Words can be poorly pronounced due to:

- Slurring (drug toxicity, alcohol ingestion)
- Mechanical problems (due to poorly fitting dentures, missing teeth (**edentulous**) or chewing gum)
- Tardive Dyskinesia

Terms used to describe this are: *garbled, slurred, mumbled, clipped, choppy, unclear,* or *poor diction.*

(IV) Modulation is the loudness or softness of speech. Some patients are naturally louder when they speak, while others add emphasis at various points in the interview. Conditions where patients speak louder than normal include:

- Mania
- Psychosis (of any cause)
- Cluster B Personality Disorders
- Dementia

Conditions where modulation is reduced include:

- Depression
- Personality disorders (e.g. avoidant, schizoid)
- Medical disorders
- Substance intoxication or withdrawal

(V) Pitch, as in music, refers to the highness or lowness of spoken words. Pitch usually varies throughout the course of a sentence. For example, it rises when questions are asked and falls when authoritative statements are made. Pitch also changes with emotional state (e.g. rising with anxiety and falling with depression). In adulthood, pitch changes occur due to throat diseases, smoking, etc. Of interest is the fact that pitch range can be altered by psychiatric illnesses (e.g. psychotic and dissociative disorders).

(VI) Spontaneity is the degree of engagement in the interview. Information volunteered without a question being posed is called *spontaneous speech*. **Latency** refers to the time interval to answer questions or connect sentences.

(VII) Rhythm, or **cadence**, varies in normal speech to add emphasis and maintain interest. Certain types of rhythm disturbances exist:

> • **Stuttering** — repetition of certain syllables
> • **Cluttering** — a nonfluent disruption involving bursts of rapid speech containing syntactical errors; the articulation is poor and the speaker is unaware of the speech abnormalities
> • **Scanning speech** — a nonfluent abnormality where there are irregular pauses between syllables, as if each one was "scanned" separately prior to being pronounced
> • **Inflection**, or stress, adds an extra communicative element to speech, contributing to the pragmatics of language

Patients with **aprosodias** miss the finer messages conveyed with stresses in speech. In many instances, non-native speakers, patients with subnormal intelligence, and those who are concrete in their thinking also miss the meanings conveyed by inflection. These situations do not constitute aprosodias.

6/ Thought Form or Process

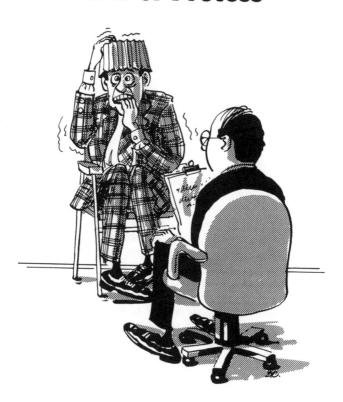

What is Thought Form/ Process?

Speech

Thought Process   **Thought Content**

Language

Speech refers to any form of verbal expression. With aphasias, speech is produced with deficits in fluency, repetition, comprehension, prosody, etc.

Language is the exchange of comprehensible ideas and describes the communicative value of speech.

Thought content describes *what* is being talked about. This is covered in detail in the next chapter.

Thought process or **thought form** refers to the way in which ideas are produced and organized. This is an assessment of *how* patients are communicating. The degree of connection and the flow of thought are disrupted in many psychiatric illnesses. When this occurs, it is referred to as a **thought disorder**. The way ideas are linked together is as important as their content. Because thought cannot be accessed directly, it is assessed via speech, writing, and behavior.

What Constitutes A Disorder of Thought Form?

The following parameters describe thought process:
- Goal directedness
- Tightness of associations between words, phrases, sentences, and paragraphs
- Rate, pressure & rhythm
- Idiosyncrasy of word usage

Thought process is easiest to assess when patients are given open-ended questions. Here, they must decide:

- What is important to say
- How directly they will answer questions
- How much detail to give, and when to move on
- How to move on to another topic, and the degree of connectedness to what was just being discussed

In a closed-ended style of interview, disorders of thought process may not be elicited. Once it is apparent that a thought disorder is present, greater structure in an interview may be the only way of moving on to salient areas. The individual disorders of thought process (listed in increasing severity) are:

- **Circumstantiality** (Section I)
- **Tangentiality** (II)
- **Flight of Ideas** (III)
- **Rambling** (IV)
- **Loose Associations** (V)
- **Thought Blocking** (VIa)
- **Thought Derailment** (VIb)
- **Fragmentation** (VII)
- **Verbigeration** (VIII)
- **Jargon** (IX)
- **Word Salad** (X)
- **Incoherence** (XI)

Process Disturbance	Nature of Disturbance
Circumstantiality **Tangentiality**	• linkage between ideas is tight • sentence structure is maintained • overinclusive of detail (circumstantiality), or does not address the point (tangentiality)

Flight of Ideas	• words and sentences maintained • connection between ideas apparent • rapid and frequent shifts in topic
Rambling	• clusters of sentences remain goal directed, but are interspersed with groups that are not goal-directed
Loose Associations	• words and sentences maintained • phrases and sentences still properly constructed • connection between ideas is not obvious, unclear, or nonsensical
Thought Blocking **Thought Derailment**	• syntax intact, but speech suddenly shifts (derailment) or halts (blocking) • patients may or may not return to the previous topic, and are unaware of what has happened
Fragmentation	• words intact but phrases become disconnected from each other
Verbigeration	• repetition of words and phrases
Jargon	• syntax intact but speech becomes meaningless
Word Salad	• words remain intact but all syntax is lost
Incoherence	• words are unintelligible, speech is garbled or dysarthric

What Is Considered Normal When It Comes to Thought Process?

People express varying degrees of coherence, detail, and organization at different times. Thought process must be considered in conjunction with other features of the interview. Someone who is overly anxious may speak quickly and provide a lot of extraneous detail. A person who is highly creative may verbalize their flow of thought ("stream of consciousness") and appear to have disjointed ideas. Some people make great leaps in thinking before verbalizing anything, and the connections between their statements may need to be explained. It is valuable to record segments of the interview to illustrate your opinion of the patient's thought process. At the end of the interview, make a judgment about the overall ability of the patient to communicate his or her difficulties. The following descriptions are commonly used:

• **Tightness of thought**
well-organized, tangential, loosely connected, or *incoherent*

• **Flow of speech**
spontaneous, hesitant, interrupted, or *halting*

• **Directness of responses**
informative and relevant, embellished, or *overinclusive*

• **Flow of ideas**
logical and with variability, restricted, or *repetitive*

• **Vocabulary**
descriptive, restricted, or *idiosyncratic use of words*

• **Flow of information**
good exchange, adequate, vague, or *disorganized*

The Mental Status Exam — Explained

Thought is normally goal-directed. In order to visualize the various disorders of thought process, the following representation will be used:

A·B·C·D·E·F·G·H·I·J·K·L·M·N·O·P·Q·R·S·T·U·V·W·X·Y·Z

where:
• Each letter represents a word
• The alphabetical sequence indicates proper syntax
• Progression from left to right indicates a logical sequence

The following propaganda statement can be schematized using the above substitution of letters.

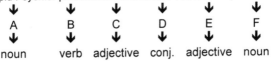

Rapid	Psychler	produces	humorous	and	educational	publications.
↓	↓	↓	↓	↓	↓
A	B	C	D	E	F
↓	↓	↓	↓	↓	↓
noun	verb	adjective	conj.	adjective	noun

A thought process disorder brings about substitution with incorrect words, though the syntax remains correct.

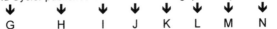

Rapid	Cycler	publishes	books	about	making	quick	bicycle	repairs.
↓	↓	↓	↓	↓	↓	↓	↓
G	H	I	J	K	L	M	N

Here, the words have different letter designations because they are different than those in the original statement. Since the grammar is correct, the letters are in alphabetical sequence. In another example of a thought disorder, a sentence that doesn't follow the rules of grammar appears as follows:

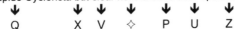

Rapido	Cyclerista	but	clear	hofic	around	then	upward.
↓		↓	↓	↓	↓	↓	↓
Q		X	V	◇	P	U	Z

Because 'hofic' isn't a word, it was represented by a symbol (neologisms are explained in detail later in this chapter).

(I) Circumstantial speech contains an overly detailed amount of information that provides a lot of digressive, extraneous detail in order to give everyone within listening distance a firm grasp on all the relevant or even quasi-relevant factors so that the point, when reached, is clearly made with substantive evidence. The preceding sentence is an example of circumstantiality. It could just as easily be defined as speech that contains an excessive amount of detail but does finally reach the point.

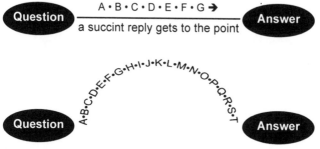

Circumstantiality involves understandable words used in a proper grammatical sequence, but with unnecessary detail. The key feature is that the point is finally made or the question answered. Circumstantiality is most commonly seen in:

- Normal conversations; it is endemic in digressive professors, politicians and most lawyers
- Obsessive-compulsive/narcissistic personalities
- Temporal lobe epilepsy
- Hypomania
- Anxiety disorders
- Substance ingestion

(II) Tangential thought remains logical and the direction can be followed. Proper words and grammar are used. The distinguishing factor is that the person does not make a point or answer your question. Tangentiality may help move a conversation along, but in an interview situation it can be a sign of pathology. The severity and frequency of tangential speech needs to be gauged to determine if it impacts on the quality of the interview. Tangential replies often stay in the "ballpark" of the answer. Patients in whom tangentiality is not pathological can refocus their replies to the question at hand when .

Example: Where did you buy your car?
My car has 4 cylinders. It gives me good gas mileage in the city but not much passing power on the highway. I live near a highway and have a garage for my car. I keep it inside even in the summer because strong sunlight makes the paint fade.

Tangential thinking is most commonly seen in:

> • Personality disorders where verbal communication is maintained principally for the sake of feeling connected to someone, e.g. histrionic and dependent personalities
> • Cognitive disorders such as delirium or dementia
> • Hypomania
> • Anxiety disorders
> • Substance ingestion and abuse (alcohol, stimulants, marijuana, etc.)
> • Schizophrenia; though other disorders of thought process are more typical of this illness

(III) Flight of ideas is non-goal directed speech that "takes off" from the topic at hand. Patients are usually distractible, and change the topic every sentence or two. Speech remains logical, and the connections between ideas are still recognizable. Patients don't elaborate on their ideas before moving onto another topic. Their statements contain proper words and grammar. Flight of ideas differs from tangential speech in that topic changes are more abrupt, more frequent, and often prompted by a word in a previous sentence.

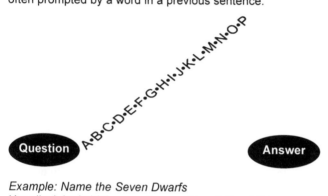

Example: Name the Seven Dwarfs
Happily, I don't think on such a small level. Small things come in good packages. I cut myself opening my mail yesterday, it still stings. I got stung by a bee last summer, but it's only fair, since I eat honey. I have breakfast every morning because it is the most important meal of the day. I like to eat three squares when I can, but not out of the can. Cans keep food around for years, but not if you take the label off. I bought a labeling machine, and now everything in my house has a proper name. I like to address my property on a first name basis. Ah, the joys of ownership!

An examination of these sentences reveals discernible connections between them, with a word acting as a trigger for the abrupt and frequent changes in topic.

Happily, I don't think on such a small level.

small

Small things come in good packages.

packages

I cut myself opening my mail yesterday,
it still stings.

sting

I got stung by a bee last summer,
but it's only fair, since I eat honey.

eating

I have breakfast every morning because
it is the most important meal of the day.

eating

I like to eat three squares when I can,
but not out of the can.

cans

Cans keep food around for years,
but not if you take the label off.

Flight of ideas is most commonly seen in:

- Mania and hypomania; flight of ideas with pressured speech is one of the cardinal signs of a manic episode
- In severe mania, patients speak in an uninterruptible monologue and head off on irrelevant tangents
- Patients often pick up on something around them to start their flight of thought; in this example, "happily" was a partial answer to the question, since Happy is one of the Seven Dwarfs
- Flight of ideas can also be seen in psychotic disorders (e.g. schizophrenia, brief psychotic disorder, drug induced psychosis), delirium, and dementia

(IV) Rambling describes speech composed of clusters of related sentences that are goal directed, but then become interspersed with loosely associated statements. It is characteristic of an acute, coarse (non-localized) brain disorder. Rambling is not as severe as loosening of associations, but lacks the discernable connections seen in flight of ideas.

(V) Loose Associations

Association refers to the logical connection or "tightness" between ideas. In loose associations, a disintegration of meaningful connections between ideas occurs. Proper words, phrases, and sentences are still used. Eugene Bleuler outlined four terms that started with 'A' as cardinal symptoms of schizophrenia. They are affective flattening, autism, ambivalence, and disturbances of association.

Example:

If the example paragraph that illustrated flight of ideas is used with every second sentence deleted (and some further editing), the following series of statements remain:

Happily, I don't think on such a small level.

?

I cut myself opening my mail yesterday.

?

I have breakfast every morning.

?

Cans keep food around for years.

?

I address my property personally.

There is no logical connection between these sentences. Loosening of associations is characteristic of the thought process during psychosis. However, mania can also become so severe that the connections between ideas is lost.

A Comparison of Thought Process Disorders

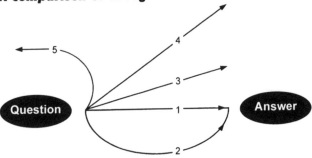

1. Goal-directed logical thought that both addresses the point and answers the question directly.

2. Circumstantial thought contains a mass of digressions, subsidiary clauses, and "talking around" the point. People are sometimes aware of their wordiness, and that their style of speech (thought) impedes reaching the goal directly.

3. Tangential thought is not goal directed, though it starts out being relevant and generally stays in the vicinity of the topic. The point or question is not ultimately addressed, which distinguishes this from circumstantiality. If the thought process does not reach the goal and is overly detailed, it can be described as both tangential and circumstantial.

4. Flight of ideas takes off more quickly and radically than tangential speech. Rapid, uncensored associations are made due to increased distractibility and the pressure to keep talking. This is a form of accelerated speech.

5. Loosening of associations is the loss of meaningful connections between words and phrases. Transitions in topic are not based on logical connections between ideas.

(VIa) Thought blocking is the sudden involuntary interruption of thought (and speech). It is not the same experience as requiring more time to formulate an idea, or being too emotionally overwhelmed to continue. Thought blocking is described as having an idea removed from consciousness or losing one's train of thought. A similar interruption in thinking and movement occurs during petit mal (absence) seizures. Thought blocking is one of the negative symptoms of schizophrenia, and is considered a form of **alogia**.

(VIb) Derailment occurs when speech begins again after an episode of thought blocking. Patients usually begin talking again after a few seconds, and on a different topic. Patients do not usually know what they were speaking about before the block, and are unaware of the change in topic. Their speech is otherwise fluent and is grammatically correct. Thought derailment is one of the positive symptoms of schizophrenia, and is considered one of the factors constituting a **formal thought disorder**.

A·B·C·D·E·F·G·H·I·J

B
L
O
C
K
I
N
G

K·L·M·N·O·P·Q·R·S·T

DERAILMENT

Example: How about those Orioles?
I think they're the team this year! They made some important changes . . . . . . I've got to catch a midnight train to Georgia.

(VII) Fragmentation is the loss of meaningful connections between words and phrases. Fragmented speech lacks focus, consisting mainly of phrases that are unrelated. The phrases themselves still have proper syntax and are composed of understandable words. This type of abnormality is similar to Broca's Aphasia in its broken delivery. However, in fragmentation, the speech contains the connecting words, articulation is intact, and pauses are not notably long.

A•B•C•D•E . . . I•J•K . . . O•P•Q•R•S•T . . . Y•Z

Example:
I have to . . . what is my . . . gone today . . . near and far . . . all or nothing at all . . . flip, flop and fly . . . whiter shade of pale

Fragmentation is not specific for any particular condition. It can be seen in psychotic disorders, mood disorders with psychotic features, dementia, delirium, etc.

(VIII) Verbigeration, also known as **palilalia**, is the automatic repetition of words or sounds. The tightness of associations in the speech may otherwise be intact.

A•B•C•C•C•C . . . . B•C•C•C•C . . . .

Example: Where did you park you car?
I parked it, it, it, it . . . . . parked it, it, it, it

This is most commonly seen in catatonia (due to schizophrenia, mood disorders, and organic brain syndromes).

(IX) Jargon, also called **jargon agrammatism** or **driveling**, is composed of speech that has lost its communicative value. The syntax is preserved in this disorder and speech remains fluent. The repetition of phrases (perseveration) or syllables (verbigeration) is not prominent.

A·C·D·C . . . U·W·O . . . P·E·X·D·U·R·P·L·E . . .

Example: What was McMaster Medical School like?
In verbatim, try delayed transparency. Principles fourth at one.

This is most commonly seen in:

  • Any of the causes of Wernicke's Aphasia (e.g.
    strokes, tumors, head injuries)
  • Chronic psychotic conditions with a severe course

(X) Word salad is an extreme form of loosened associations
to the point that words have no connection to one another.
The speech in word salad is incomprehensible, and resembles
the incoherence of a **global aphasia**. The articulation remains
intact, delivery is usually fluent and the prosody of speech is
present.

Word salad differs from fragmentation in that in word salad
there is no connection between individual words. Recall that
in **fragmentation** the phrases and sentences are uncon-
nected. Word salad differs from **jargon** in that in word salad
there is no preservation of syntax, though the speech in both
disorders is meaningless.

A·X·Q·D·B·E·B·O·P·A·O·L·S·U·X·P·O·R·V·T·X·X·W·V·T·Z

Example: So, what are those secret herbs and spices?
at, to, but, not, when, if, that, my, never, fuller, clip.

This is most commonly seen in:

  • Chronic schizophrenia (with a severe course)
  • Advanced dementias
  • Severe delirium.

(XI) Incoherence (unintelligible, garbled speech) can be caused by:

- Severe dysarthria
- Extensive use of made-up words (neologisms)
- Private use of words (words that exist but are used in an incorrect way)

Other Disorders of Thought Process

- **Punning** (XII)
- **Clang Associations** (XIII)
- **Echolalia** (XIV)
- **Perseveration** (XV)
- **Neologisms** (XVI)
- **Non sequiturs** (XVII)
- **Private use of words** (XVIII)
- **Rate abnormalities** (XIX)

(XII) A pun is a play on words which is made humorous by involving double meanings or similar sounding-words:

- Santa's helpers are subordinate clauses.
- Buddhist to a hot dog vendor: "Make me one with everything."

Continual punning can be a disorder of thought process. Some patients are compelled to use words for their sounds or alternate meanings (such as homonyms). In flight of ideas, the connections between words or ideas may be based on their multiple or abstract meanings.

(XIII) Clang associations are made on the basis of sound, not syntax or logical flow. This occurs most commonly by rhyming the last word in a sentence. In some cases, this is considered a type of **phonemic** or **literal paraphasia** where patients substitute a word that sounds similar to one they just used, for example:

"I have to go, you know. To and fro before the snow blows."

Clang associations are most commonly seen in mania, but also occur in aphasias, schizophrenia, and dementias.

(XIV) Echolalia has been mentioned earlier in the Behavior Chapter. It is the automatic repetition of someone else's speech. Echolalia is seen in:

- Catatonia
- Transcortical motor and sensory aphasias
- Dementias

Echolalia is distinguished from **perseveration** in that the words repeated are the interviewer's (not the patient's as in perseveration). Echolalia is distinguished from **palilalia** (**verbigeration**) in that whole phrases and sentences are repeated, not just the last word or syllable.

(XV) Perseveration is the automatic repetition of a verbal response despite changing questions. Perseveration can also be a motor disorder where the same action persists. The repeated group of words is called a **stock phrase**.

C . . . C . . . C . . . C . . . C . . . C . . . C . . . C

Example: Where did you park your car?
Garage.
How long have you been in town?
Garage.
Where should the hospital administrator's office go?
Garage.

Perseveration is most commonly seen in: mood disorders, schizophrenia, catatonia, and frontal lobe damage.

(XVI) Neologisms are words or phrases made up by patients that have idiosyncratic meanings for them. Neologisms may be formed by the improper use of word sounds or other perceptual abnormalities. They are also called **jargon paraphasias**. In psychiatric disorders, neologisms occur in syntactically correct places, as if they are words the interviewer should know. Ask patients about unfamiliar terms — you'll either detect a neologism or learn a new word! Additionally, neologisms sound as if they could be words. For example, which in the following list are actual words?

- jolmet
- jingo
- meltom
- monad

The first and third words are neologisms that have meanings that only a patient using them would understand. Jolmet might be the border surrounding a sheet of stamps; meltom could be the ground on an electrical plug. No sense can be made of these words by breaking them down into their components.

Neologisms can appear in any of the disorders of thought form listed in this chapter. They are most commonly seen in schizophrenia, but can occur in any type of psychotic disorder, dementia, and several of the aphasias. Patients are not generally aware that they have used a neologism, and are usually cooperative in defining the term once its use has been pointed out.

(XVII) Non-sequitur is a Latin term meaning *does not follow*. Non-sequiturs occur readily in normal speech and thought. If someone gets an idea or is suddenly reminded of something (e.g. Got milk?), he or she may blurt out something apart from what was just being discussed. The reply itself demonstrates proper grammar and syntax, and except for not addressing the question, it is not otherwise remarkable.

Non-sequiturs can also be a sign of pathology. Generally, they are considered to occur whenever the answer given is unrelated to the question that was posed.

(XVIII) Private use of words refers to the incorrect use of an existing word. Syntax remains correct, but the word is used out of context. It is also called a **literal** or **semantic paraphasia**. The word substituted for the correct one is unrelated either in sound or function. For example, "*Yesterday I visited my friend gerund.*" Gerund is a word, but its use here is of a private nature. It was not substituted for Gerrard, which would have been either a related (approximative) or literal (phonemic) aphasia.

(XIX) Rate Abnormalities

The **rate** of speech, or more correctly the rate of thought, constitutes another disorder of thought process. A rapid rate of speech may be a variant of normal, and is frequently seen when patients are anxious (either situational or due to an anxiety disorder).

Pressured speech has a rapid rate with an uninterruptible, intrusive quality, as if patients are compelled to keep talking. This is also called **pressure of ideas** or **thought pressure**.

At an average rate, reading this sentence takes about 3 seconds —

Rapid Psychler produces humorous and educational publications.

Pressured speech takes less time and keeps going (and going) —

Rapid Psychler produces humorous and educational publications. Using humor is a key component in making material interesting. . .

Pressure of speech is one of the principal signs of a manic episode, and is accompanied by the sensation of **racing thoughts**. The combination of pressured speech and racing thought is expressed verbally as **flight of ideas**. These features can also occur in anxiety states, use of stimulants, and hyperthyroidism. Rate of speech (and thought) varies widely in psychiatric illnesses. Rate tends to vary with amount of speech and loudness. In mania, patients speak quickly, have a lot to say, and say it loudly. Depressed patients speak in the opposite manner. Increased rate needs to be distinguished from pressure of speech. Patients who have a rapid rate of speech are interruptible, do not appear compelled to keep speaking, and may be anxious. When asked to do so, they are able to slow their rate of speech.

Thought Process Practice Points
• It can be quite difficult to distinguish **word salad** from **Wernicke's Aphasia**

• If the associations between someone's thoughts seem loosened, point out the shift in topic to the patient and ask what the connection is between the two ideas

• Patients demonstrate loosening of associations when writing as well as speaking

• Although loose associations are considered a cardinal sign of schizophrenia, they are also seen in cognitive disorders (delirium & depression), mood disorders (especially severe mania or psychotic depression), and drug intoxication or withdrawal states.

• **Thought insertion** or **thought withdrawal** can affect the process of thought by increasing or decreasing (respectively) the number of ideas to express

• **Condensation** is a disorder of thought process in which several concepts are expressed in a unified form; this occurs mainly in schizophrenia and substance abuse

Psychiatric vs. Neurologic Terminology

Psychspeak	Neurospeak
Driveling speech	Jargon agrammatism
Neologisms	Phonemic paraphasias
Private use of words	Semantic paraphasias
Verbigeration	Palilalia

Thought Process Disorder vs. Aphasia

A thought process disorder generally doesn't interfere with:

- Reading
- Writing
- Copying
- Naming
- Repeating

In thought process disorders, neologisms are symbolic (replace a noun or verb), repeated, and used in a syntactically correct way. In aphasias, they can replace any word (nonsymbolic), are not repeated, and occur randomly. Aphasias cause the deletion of connecting words (articles, prepositions, conjunctions, etc.), so speech consists mainly of nouns and verbs. Patients with thought disorders generally speak fluently with preserved syntax and prosody.

7/ Thought Content

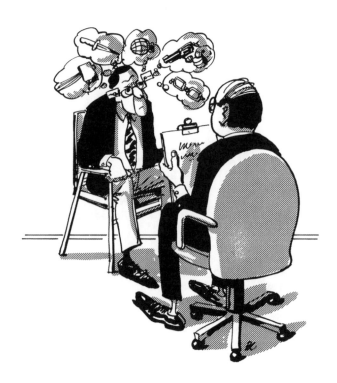

Thought content refers to *what* patients talk about in the course of the interview. While it may be tempting to say, "Ms. C.Y. answered the questions I asked her," interviews are strongly influenced by the content of the patients' answers.

One of the key reasons that the first few minutes of an interview is left relatively unstructured is to allow for an assessment of the patient's thought content. Special attention should be given to what topics patients talk about spontaneously, elaborate on, and what themes develop.

As stressors or symptoms are elicited, exploration helps guide the flow of relevant material, while also allowing patients the chance to continue speaking in a relatively unrestricted manner. Interviews that consist of a closed-ended or "laundry list" approach restrict the flow of spontaneous information.

What Constitutes A Disorder of Thought Content?

Thought content is considered abnormal when it contains the following elements:

- **Delusions** (Section I)
    - paranoid
    - grandiose
    - jealous
    - erotomanic
    - somatic
    - passivity and control

- **Overvalued Ideas** (II)
- **Obsessions** (III)
- **Phobias** (IV)
- **Thoughts of Harm to Self or Others** (V)

Patients experiencing delusions, obsessions or phobias seek attention because their lives, or the lives of those around them, are significantly disrupted by these disturbances in thought content. On the other hand, some patients are adept at concealing such experiences and make them difficult to elicit, especially during a first interview. The degree of awareness of abnormal thoughts (**insight**) varies widely. Impaired or absent insight is usually a sign of a more serious disturbance and/or a worse prognosis. Additionally, abnormal thoughts evoke variable emotional responses from patients.

(I) Delusions are one of the cardinal symptoms indicating a serious mental illness, though they have been reported to occur in well over fifty psychiatric and general medical conditions. A delusion is defined as a fixed, false belief that:

- Is inconsistent with cultural or subcultural norms
- Is inappropriate for the person's level of education
- Is not altered with proof to the contrary
- Preoccupies the thoughts of the patient
- Is not resisted by the patient
- Ranges from implausible to impossible

The content of delusions ranges from fragmented to systematized, and from situations that are possible (**non-bizarre**) to those that are impossible (**bizarre**). In cases where a patient appears to have a discrete, plausible, but false belief (e.g. "someone reads my mail"), it may only be possible to establish the presence of a delusion when collateral information becomes available. Cultural differences can also account for unusual ideas. In order to distinguish a delusion from other aberrations of thought content, it is crucial to establish that it is indeed fixed. For example, someone who is confabulating (or is being misleading) will quite likely change some part of the history when asked to repeat the details.

Delusions that start *de novo* are called **primary delusions**. **Secondary delusions** arise out of a mood state, perceptual abnormality (including sensory deprivation or impairment), social factors, or other pre-existing psychopathology.

Delusional patients demonstrate altered reasoning processes. **Apophony** (from the Greek "to become manifest") is the phenomenon in which arbitrary or false ideas are considered fact without adequate proof. This is also called **delusional intuition**. Events and objects become imbued with a personal, autistic significance.

Delusional patients make sweeping inferences based on small amounts of information (the process of **generalization**). They do not use their knowledge or experience to modify their beliefs. For example, a patient who passes through a radar trap (without speeding) would become convinced that "surveillance" was arranged so the police could monitor his or her actions. Delusions become a psychological compromise, and help to make sense of the internal chaos with which patients must contend (a process called **consolidation**).

How Do I Ask About Delusions?

Formulating questions about delusions constitutes one of the most difficult interviewing tasks. As opposed to patients with phobias or obsessions, delusional patients usually don't recognize that they are ill. Asking, "So, are you delusional?" probably won't work, necessitating a more refined approach.

1. Look for themes during the interview.
Despite the complexity of mental illnesses, most delusions fall into a small number of themes (paranoid, somatic, grandiose, jealous, and erotomanic).

2. Questions to help detect the presence of delusions:

- *"Do you spend a lot of time thinking about one or two things?"*
- *"Do you have some ideas that you hold very strongly?"*
- *"Do others frequently disagree with your views on things?"*
- *"What are the things that are most important to you?"*

Because delusions dominate patients' thoughts, these questions are likely to reveal an aspect of delusional thinking if it is present. When patients mention something that could be of a delusional nature, respond with curiosity. An interested, conversational manner will elicit more information.

3. Questions to explore delusional material:

- *"How do you know (that this is going on)?"*
- *"How did this situation start?"*
- *"Why would someone want to do this to you?"*
- *"How do you account for what has happened?"*

Regardless of interviewer skill, delusions can't always be elicited. Patients with an awareness that others don't share their ideas (preserved insight), or who have been hospitalized because of delusional thinking may conceal their ideas.

Mood Congruence & Ego Syntonicity

The terms **mood-congruent** and **mood-incongruent** are applied to delusions and hallucinations (which are psychotic features) that occur with mood disorders. Themes of guilt, worthlessness, death, failure, hopelessness, punishment, illness, etc. are congruent to feeling depressed. If the content of delusions expressed by depressed patients is along these lines, the term *mood-congruent* is applicable.

In manic episodes, mood-congruent delusions involve themes of power, brilliance, wealth, longevity, achievement, special relationships or connections, knowledge, etc.

Manic patients with delusions of nihilism, poverty or inadequacy have *mood-incongruent delusions*, as would depressed patients with delusions of grandeur, omnipotence or connections to famous people. Mood-incongruent delusions are a poor prognostic sign, and may indicate that a schizoaffective or schizophreniform disorder is present.

The term **egosyntonic** is used to refer to symptoms that are not foreign or distressing to patients. Patients do not experience delusional thoughts as disturbing. The delusional beliefs become accepted as reality, and are therefore egosyntonic. For example, paranoid patients are not disturbed by experiencing continual thoughts of persecution. Instead, they accept that the world is this way, and are ever vigilant for evidence to confirm that they are being conspired against.

(II) Overvalued ideas differ from delusions in that they are less firmly held, and their content is often less absurd. Beliefs become *overvalued* in that they preoccupy the patient's thinking, and alter behavior. Examples of overvalued ideas are *superstitions* or *magical thinking*. A superstitious (as opposed to delusional) patient will concede that walking under a ladder isn't *really* likely to change his luck, but he feels better not doing such things. Situations where delusions seem probable but are not clearly present are recorded as overvalued ideas.

(III) Obsessions are thoughts, impulses, or images that are:

- Recurrent and persistent
- Unwanted (called **ego-alien** or **egodystonic**)
- Not simply an exaggerated degree of concern over current problems
- Recognized as a product of the patient's own mind; obsessions are generated from *within* as opposed to from *without* (as in **thought insertion**)
- Not able to be controlled by the person's will

• Recognized as absurd and irrational
• Resisted, at least at some point to some degree

Obsessive Themes

Like delusions, obsessions tend to fall into a relatively small number of themes:

Theme	Obsession
Cleanliness	Contamination
Order	Symmetry, Precision
Sex & Aggression	Assault, Sexual Assault, Homicide, Insults
Doubt	Safety, Catastrophe Unworthiness

How Do I Ask About Obsessions?

Obsessions are recognized by patients as absurd and distressing, yet they are not expressed as dominantly in interviews as are delusions. Suggestions for inquiries are:

• *Do you experience repetitive thoughts that you can't stop?*
• *Do they feel like your own thoughts?*
• *Are you ever forced to think something against your will?*

Preoccupations are another component of thought content; they differ from obsessions in that they are a willful return to thinking or conversing about a topic. **Ruminations** are another term for intellectual obsessions; here, people "chew" (mull over) their "cud" (thoughts), but reach no resolution. There is an irritating and unnecessary quality (both in time and degree) to this type of thought, which is often a manifestation of ambivalence.

(IV) Phobias are marked and persistent fears that are:

• Viewed by the patient as excessive and unreasonable (phobias are **egodystonic**)
• Clearly circumscribed (the person has clearly demarcated objects or situations that are feared)
• Accompanied by a sense of anxiety upon exposure or the thought of exposure to the object(s) or situation(s)
• Capable of causing sufficient distress so that patients go to great lengths to avoid the anxiety-provoking stimulus
• Of generally benign objects or situations; for example, fears of a rabid Doberman or a dangerous neighborhood are justified; fear of numbers is not

Categories of specific phobias and social phobias can be recalled with the following mnemonic:

"ASP & BOAS"

Animal type — e.g. killer Chihuahuas
Situational type — e.g. bridges, tunnels, flying, etc.
People (social phobia) — e.g. public speaking

Blood/Injection
Other — used when other categories won't do
Agoraphobia — avoidance of places where escape
    or getting help are difficult
Surroundings — elements in the natural environment
    such as storms, water, heights, etc.

Agoraphobia is a condition that deserves special mention. The word is derived from Greek and means "fear of the marketplace." The DSM-IV defines it as: *anxiety about being in places or situations from which escape might be difficult (or embarrassing) or in which help may not be available in the event of having an unexpected or situationally predisposed panic attack or panic-like symptoms.*

Agoraphobia is a common phobia, and the one that causes the greatest impairment of social and occupational functioning. Generally, patients who experience repeated panic attacks become "phobic" of the places where attacks occur, or in situations where help or escape would be difficult to arrange. Patients who have a moderate/severe course of panic disorder frequently have some degree of agoraphobia. Patients with agoraphobia make constant demands on friends and family members to accompany them on outings. They frequently need to be seated near the exit on a bus or in a movie theater. Patients can become housebound if others cannot oblige their requests or if the illness becomes too severe.

How Do I Ask About Phobias?

Phobias are not usually difficult to ask about because they are egodystonic, and patients recognize them as excessive. Unless patients have agoraphobia or fear something in the room, phobias are not likely cause anxiety during the interview. The presence of phobias can also be inferred through behavior. For example, someone who avoids the public acceptance of an award may have a social phobia or agoraphobia. Suggestions for questions to screen for the presence of phobias are as follows:

Specific Phobias:
• *Are there objects or situations that make you intensely anxious if you cannot avoid them?*
• *Do you make special efforts to avoid certain objects or situations?*

Social Phobias:
• *Do you have strong or persistent fears about being humiliated in public?*
• *Do you have strong or persistent fears that you will do something embarrassing in front of strangers?*

Agoraphobia:
• *Do you require special arrangements to be made for you to be comfortable when outside your home?*
• *Do you have such a strong sense of anxiety that someone must be with you before you can leave your house?*

(V) Thoughts of Harm to Self or Others
The following mnemonic covers the key elements in assessing suicidal risk:

"SADDLE SORE WOMAN"

Social isolation
Age
Disturbed interpersonal relationships (DIRs)
Drug use/abuse
Lethality of method
Ethanol use

Sex (gender)
Occupation
Repeated attempts
Event — acute precipitant

Will — created or altered
Organic condition — chronic medical illness
Mental illness
Antidepressant use
Note written

Another important factor is **family history**. There are studies that demonstrate a genetic inheritance for suicide risk independent of other major risk factors (mood disorders, schizophrenia, and alcoholism). Patients who have lost parents to suicide may not only suffer from **anniversary reactions**, but may also be involved unconsciously in a self-destructive process at the same age as the parent who died. In our individualized and technological society, the cumulative weight of moderate stressors can be too much for some people. Some of the most difficult stressors are:

- Death of a spouse or a family member
- Divorce/separation
- Serious medical illness
- Being fired or retiring from work

Conditions Associated With Violence
"MADS & BADS"

Mania (due to high energy level and poor judgment)
Alcohol (intoxication or withdrawal)
Dementia
Schizophrenia (especially the paranoid subtype)

Borderline Personality Disorder — intense anger
Antisocial Personality Disorder — disregard for safety
Delirium — hallucinations and delusions
Substance Abuse — hallucinogens, PCP

Factors Increasing the Risk of Violence
"ARM PAIN"

Altered state of consciousness — delirium
Repeated assaults — history of violence
Male gender

Paranoia (schizophrenia, mania, delusional disorder)
Age — more likely to be violent if younger
Incapacity — brain injury, psychosis, etc.
Neurologic disease

8/ Affect & Mood

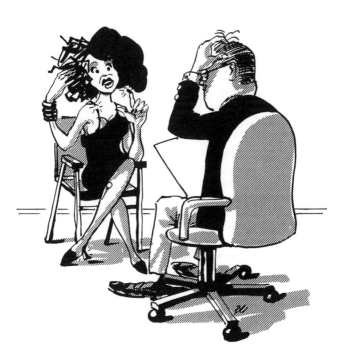

Affect refers to the visible, external or objective manifestations of a patient's emotional state. It is a record of the momentary dynamic changes in the expression of emotional responses. Both internal (e.g. memories, ideas) and external events (e.g. aspects of the environment) can change affect.

Mood is the person's internal feeling state. It is described by the patient (subjective), and refers to the pervasive emotional tone displayed throughout the interview. Mood changes are less connected to internal or external stimuli, and occur less spontaneously. Mood is considered the "emotional background" whereas affect is the "emotional foreground" of the interview. Affect can be likened to one's degree of satisfaction with the various courses of a meal, while mood is the overall enjoyment of the entire evening.

What Are the Various Aspects of Affect?

- **Type/Quality** (Section I)
- **Range/Variability** (II)
- **Degree/Intensity** (III)
- **Stability** (IVa) **Reactivity** (IVb)
- **Appropriateness** (V)
- **Congruence** (VI)
     to Mood (VIa)
     to Appearance (VIb)
     to Behavior (VIc)

(I) Type or **quality** is the predominant emotion expressed. There are nine principal types of affect:

- Happiness
- Surprise
- Interest
- Sadness
- Shame
- Disgust
- Fear/Anxiety
- Anger
- Contentment

(II) Range refers to the degree to which visible emotions vary throughout the interview. During the assessment, a patient's "normal" affective tone would consist of a combination of a number of the emotional qualities listed in section (I).

At some point in the interview, a patient would be expected to smile, frown, appear interested, and show some manifestation of emotion. A *narrow* or *restricted* range of affect describes patients who express one or two emotional states. This can be seen in mood disorders (manic patients can have a narrowly high range), schizophrenia, paranoid disorders, and obsessive-compulsive personalities. A *wide* or *expanded* range, where several emotions are expressed, is seen in cluster B personality disorders, dementia, and substance use.

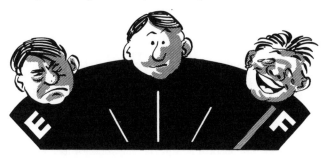

(III) Degree is the extent or **intensity** to which emotions are expressed. This can also be called **amount** or **amplitude**, and is a measure of the energy expended in conveying feelings. Affective expression occurs along a continuum:

Low Intensity	Normal	High Intensity
flattened	appropriate	exaggerated
constricted	responsive	dramatic
detached	adequate	passionate

Patients can have an intense affect with a narrow range (e.g. mania or depression). Conversely, a wide range of expression with low intensity is also seen (e.g. histrionic personalities lack a degree of depth to their affective states). **Blunted affect** is a term often used to describe low or flattened intensity. Sims (1995) uses the term to describe a lack of emotional sensitivity to others.

A flattened intensity of affect can be seen in schizophrenia, conversion disorder (**la belle indifférence**), dementia, and obsessive-compulsive and schizoid personalities. A heightened degree of affect can be seen in mania, narcissistic or borderline personalities, and anxiety disorders. Depression has a variable presentation: some patients convey intense distress while others are muted and appear apathetic.

(IVa) Stability refers to the duration of an affective response. Some emotions exist only as long as a facial expression, others are pervasive throughout the interview. Normally, there are shifts in affect during interviews. These periods are sustained for a few moments and appropriate to the context of the interview. If changes in affect are small or nonexistent during the interview (called *fixed* or *immobile*), this observation is more a description of mood. However, affect is an objective description of how the patient appears to the interviewer. The term *labile* describes affective changes that occur rapidly and frequently. These changes can take place in either the **intensity** or **range** of affect. For example, a patient may be moved from tears to euphoria within seconds (range) or from mild to intense irritation (degree).

(IVb) Reactivity of affect refers to the degree to which external factors influence emotional expression. Another parameter of lability is whether or not patients appear to be in control of their emotions. In general, patients with mood disorders, substance intoxication or withdrawal, and dementia have little to no control over their affective state. Patients with personality disorders have a greater degree of control. Lability of affect is commonly seen in the following conditions:

- Mania (affect can vary rapidly, e.g. from elated to irritable; expansive to hostile)
- Cluster B personalities (this is one of the defining aspects of histrionic and borderline personalities)
- Delirium & dementia
- Intoxication with drugs or alcohol
- Impulse Control Disorders

(V) Appropriateness is the degree to which visible emotions match thought content. This is also gauged by the degree to which you can empathize with patients. Affect is either *appropriate* or *inappropriate* to the topic being discussed. For example, a patient who smiles when discussing the death of a parent may be seen as displaying an *inappropriate* affect. If you later learn that this parent was abusive or estranged (or left a large inheritance), then this person's smile is more understandable, and the expressed emotion is more *appropriate* to the situation.

Inappropriate affect occurs most frequently in schizophrenia, which can cause patients to exhibit a detached demeanor and lose the ability to relate to others. Their emotional responses are not what would normally be expected for the topics being discussed. Patients can demonstrate what is called a *silly* or *fatuous affect*. This occurs when patients exhibit qualities such as: giggling, laughing, grinning, rhyming, punning, mocking interviewers, playing with objects, and other childlike actions. Inappropriate affect is also seen in:

- Malingering
- Conversion Disorder
- Substance use
- Depression

(VI) Congruence between affect and other factors in the MSE is another important consideration. The association between affect and the following parameters is important to observe:

(VIa) Mood
Affect may or may not be congruent to the mood state a patient reports. For example, depressed patients may still smile, joke and discuss Caribbean cruises. Lack of congruity may mean malingering or a factitious disorder, the presence of two separate conditions (e.g. a mood disorder and a personality disorder), substance use, schizoaffective disorder, or a psychotic component to a mood disorder.

(VIb) Appearance
Emotional disturbances are often manifested in various aspects of appearance because patients have little time or interest in attending to the finer points of grooming and attire. Depressed patients often neglect their self-care, are disheveled, and dress in dark colors. Manic patients dress flamboyantly and use poor judgment in picking new looks or styles. Schizophrenic patients may make bizarre alterations to their appearance and become unkempt.

(VIc) Behavior
Facial expression is a key component of affective response. Unvarying movements are seen in depression and schizophrenia; in mania and personality disorders, expressions can be overly dramatic and exaggerated.

Body movement/Gesticulation also indicates affective tone. Depressed patients move infrequently and slowly; manic patients emphasize their feelings with rapid and exaggerated movements and have trouble restraining their activities.

What Are the Various Aspects of Mood?

Mood is evaluated according to the following parameters:

- **Quality/Type** (Section VII)
- **Reactivity** (VIII)
- **Intensity** (IX)
- **Stability/ Duration** (X)

(VII) Quality of mood is the patient's reported emotional state (therefore, you must ask!). The DSM-IV includes the following as pathological mood types:

- Depressed
- Angry/Irritable
- Euphoric
- Anxious

Depressed mood occurs when patients feel less energetic, hopeful, or capable than what is usual for them. This mood state can be described by any of a number of qualifying terms, such as: *sad, blue, worthless, guilty, flat, hollow, miserable, gloomy, glum, forlorn, morose, troubled, exhausted, somber, brooding, unhappy, subdued, withdrawn, etc*. Because depression is used to refer to mood disorders, these mood states are often referred to as *dysphoric* (meaning a state of unhappiness or feeling ill at ease). Depressed mood is a diagnostic criterion for the following disorders:

- Depression
- Depressed phase of bipolar mood disorders
- Cyclothymia
- Dysthymia
- Adjustment disorder with depressed mood

The diagnosis of a mood disorder rests on associated features, severity (degree of social and occupational impairment), and duration. Major depressive episodes can be a complication of any other psychiatric condition. The term **double depression** refers to an episode of depression complicating a dysthymic disorder. Depressed mood can be such a long-standing experience for patients that it becomes a character trait. Depressed mood is often accompanied by changes in:

- Appearance (decline in self-care)
- Behavior (few spontaneous movements)
- Speech (speak softly, have little to say, etc.)
- Affect (restricted range, variable intensity)
- Thought content (morbid themes)
- Thought form (increased latency of responses)
- Diminished cognitive functioning

Euphoric mood occurs when patients feel energized, elated or ecstatic. This is of a greater degree than what is experienced when patients are "up" or in a "good mood." Some of the terms used to describe euphoric mood are: *up, flying, grand, uninhibited, omnipotent, buoyant, jovial, racing, driven, on top of the world, etc.* Euphoric mood is seen in:

- Mania/hypomania
- Schizophrenia (usually the disorganized type)
- Substance use (particularly with stimulants)
- Dementia and delirium

When patients are experiencing a dysphoric mood, they frequently seek help for the way they feel. When patients are euphoric, they rarely present for assistance and generally have to be brought to medical attention because of the impact their mood state is having on others, or on social/occupational functioning.

Angry/Irritable moods do not constitute discrete disorders, but are frequent complications of other conditions. Some of the following terms are used to describe these mood states: *annoyed, miffed, pi**ed off, seething, sharp, disgruntled, cranky, indignant, incensed, bellicose, smoldering, exasperated, furious, ill-tempered, easily provoked, etc.* These mood states frequently accompany the following conditions:

- Mania/hypomania
- Cluster B personality disorders
- Disorders where paranoia is prominent
- Substance use, particularly withdrawal syndromes
- Delirium & dementia
- Intermittent Explosive Disorder

Irritability is defined as being easily provoked to anger. The DSM-IV lists irritability as one of the three mood states seen in mania or hypomania. Irritability is usually seen as a manic or hypomanic episode increases in severity.

Anxious mood can occur normally, especially if patients are unfamiliar with or intimidated by the interview process. It is to be expected that patients will be anxious about such areas as diagnosis, prognosis, and treatment implications. Anxiety is pathological when it is pervasive or present to a degree that interferes with social or occupational functioning. Terms used to describe an anxious mood are: *fearful, tense, on edge, worried, nervous, uptight, frazzled, petrified, uneasy, rattled, terrified, paralyzed, etc.* Anxiety is prominently seen in:

- Phobic disorders
- Panic Disorder
- Generalized Anxiety Disorder
- Obsessive-Compulsive Disorder
- Posttraumatic Stress Disorder
- Adjustment Disorder with Anxiety

As with other dysphoric mood states, anxiety can complicate any other psychiatric condition and is prominent in a number of general medical conditions (hyperthyroidism, cardiac arrythmias, pheochromocytoma, etc.).

(VIII) Reactivity is the degree to which mood is altered by external factors. Mood can be shifted by events, the environment, or interactions with others. Manic patients often escalate in mood with stimulation. Depressed patients may feel worse in the morning and have their spirits lift as the day progresses. Similarly, anxious or angry patients have a waxing and waning of their mood under certain conditions.

In the past, depression was divided into **endogenous** and **reactive** types based on the presence of a (presumed) precipitant. The endogenous aspect has been carried forward into a subtype of depression called the **melancholic features specifier**. In this type of depression, there is a lack of mood reactivity to usually pleasurable stimuli. Another subtype of depression, called the **atypical features specifier**, contains two criteria related to mood reactivity:

• Mood brightening in response to actual or potentially positive events
• A long-standing pattern of interpersonal rejection sensitivity (not limited to episodes of mood disturbance) resulting in significant social or occupational impairment

Depressed patients with melancholic features have a greater likelihood of response to medication or ECT than patients without these features. Atypical features occur more frequently in women and younger patients. Frequently, only a partial recovery from these episodes is reported. Atypical features may indicate a bipolar depression or a seasonal pattern.

(IX) Intensity refers to the degree to which the mood is expressed. Like affect, mood has depth, quality, and amplitude. Two patients can experience depressed mood with a similarly flat affect and restricted range of emotional expression. One patient may appear lethargic, withdrawn, and show little interest in the interview. The other patient may have problems with concentration, lowered self-esteem, and be able to convey the degree to which this episode has interfered with his or her life. The difference between these patients is the depth or intensity of their mood state.

(X) Stability or duration describes the length of time the mood disturbance exists without significant variation. Mood disorders are required to have a specific time course:

• Major Depressive Episode	2 weeks
• Manic Episode	1 week
• Dysthymic Disorder	2 years
• Cyclothymia	2 years

How Do I Ask About Mood Symptoms?

Mood symptoms are usually distressing to patients and they speak about them or display them readily in interviews. Since mood is a subjective phenomenon, patients need to be asked about their emotional state.

• *"How have you been feeling lately?"*
• *"How would you describe your mood right now?"*
• *"I'd like you to rate your mood on a scale from 1 to 10. If 1 is the worst you've ever felt, and 10 is the best, what score would you give yourself right now?"*

Some patients will answer feeling questions with thinking answers, e.g. *"I feel that the Orioles will win the World Series"* or *"I feel like a pizza"* are not considered statements of mood.

It may be necessary to point out a patient's reactions as a means of eliciting information about mood, e.g. *"You looked very sad when you were talking about being ripped off at the drive-thru. How were you feeling at that time?"* As with affect, incongruities between reported mood state and observable signs need to be explored.

A difficulty commonly encountered in interviews is being able to distinguish mania/hypomania from the elevated mood states that most people report from time to time. The following questions may help make this distinction:

• *"Was your mood ever so high that friends or family members thought you needed to get help?"*

• *"Did you get yourself into serious financial, legal or relationship trouble when your mood was high?"*

• *"Did your mood ever become so elevated that you thought you had some supernatural powers, special connections to important people, or revolutionary ideas?"*

9/ Perception

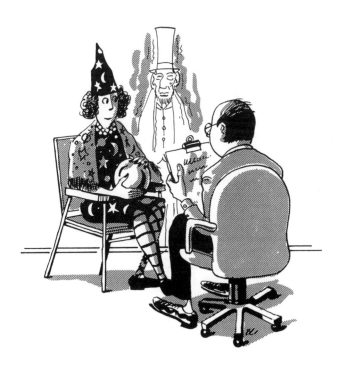

Perception is the process of experiencing the environment and recognizing or making sense of the stimuli received via sensory input. An object in the environment causes a **sensation**, which upon interpretation by the brain becomes a **perception**. Disorders of perception in psychiatry involve false associations or the *de novo* arrival of a percept without a stimulus. While imagination can bring about perceptions in any sensory modality, there is normally no difficulty in distinguishing this response from external stimuli. Patients experience perceptual abnormalities as clearly as they do reality, but have lost the ability to make a clear distinction between the two.

What Are the Various Aspects of Perception?

- **Hallucinations** (Section I)
- **Illusions** (II)
- **Disturbances of Self and Environment** (III)
  - Depersonalization
  - Derealization
- **Disturbances of Quality or Size** (IV)
  - Micropsia
  - Macropsia
  - Dysmegalopsia
- **Disturbances in the Intensity of Perception** (V)
  - Hyperacusis
  - Visual hyperaesthesia
- **Disturbances of Experience (VI)**
  - Déjà vu
  - Jamais vu

(I) Hallucinations are perceptions that occur when there is no actual stimulus present. They are the most severe of the disorders of perception. Additional features of hallucinations are that they:

- Occur in all sensory modalities

- Can be simple or complex
- Seem as vivid as real life experiences
- Occur spontaneously
- Are often intrusive (as are obsessions)
- Are internal experiences attributed to external sources

Hallucinations are given the following terms according to the sensory modalities in which they occur:

Sense	Name of Hallucination
sight	visual
sound	auditory
smell	olfactory
taste	gustatory
touch	somatic

Brief, poorly formed experiences are called **incomplete, unformed** or **elementary hallucinations**. Examples are flashes of light, whispered sounds, faint odors or tastes, or the sensation of being gently nudged.

• **Auditory Hallucinations** are the most common type in psychiatric conditions. In general, they occur as distinctly heard voices that speak clearly formed words, sentences or even conversations. In organic conditions, they are more like *elementary hallucinations*, involving indistinct sounds such as ringing, grating or humming.

Auditory hallucinations are one of the cardinal symptoms of schizophrenia, and are part of the criteria for schizophreniform disorder, schizoaffective disorder, brief psychotic disorder, and psychotic disorders due to general medical conditions. Patients are usually able to describe their "voices" in some detail. They are aware of the gender of the hallucinatory speaker and whether or not they recognize the voice. Often, it is some-one they know or someone that has passed away. In some instances, patients are instructed by a voice to perform an act; this experience is called a **command hallucination**. The repetitive nature of these commands can be too much to bear, and patients may eventually act on them.

Auditory hallucinations are usually derogatory and critical to-wards patients. Carrying around this cacophony of insulting, belittling comments is one of the tortures of mental illness. Hallucinations are one of the **positive symptoms** of schizo-phrenia, and are usually responsive to antipsychotic medica-tions. Auditory hallucinations can be of sounds other than voices. Commonly, these include: machine-like sounds, mu-sic, and animal vocalizations. Auditory hallucinations in or-ganic conditions tend not to be as distinct or have the same duration as those in psychiatric illnesses.

• **Visual Hallucinations** are the next most prevalent type en-countered in psychiatric illnesses. It is more common to have visual and auditory hallucinations occurring together than it is to have visual hallucinations alone. One such combination involves auditory hallucinations with partial or inferred visual hallucinations. For example, a patient who hears a voice com-ing from the coat rack may also see or "might have seen" arms gesturing as "it" was speaking. Isolated visual halluci-nations should prompt a thorough investigation for an organic cause (a medical condition or the effects of a substance). When visual hallucinations occur exclusively in psychiatric con-ditions, they are almost always due to a psychotic disorder. Visual hallucinations can be simple or complex. They can be as brief as a vision or as involved as having a visit from Abe Lincoln. **Extracampine Hallucinations** involve experiences beyond the normal sensory range (e.g., being able to look out the window and see someone in another state). Visual hallu-cinations can also form, or be part of, delusional thinking. A patient who experiences a raging Viking leaping out of her hospital closet may develop delusions of persecution. Paranoid patients commonly "see" their persecutors in various public places or just outside their homes.

Oneiroid States (from Greek, meaning dream-like) occur in schizophrenia and delirium. The patient experiences vivid hallucinations, which can range from terrifying to engrossing. Oneiroid states can become an alternate world. Patients can keep track of oneiroid states and reality at the same time

The **Charles Bonnet Syndrome** is a rare condition consisting of formed, complex, repetitive visual hallucinations (that are recognized as such). There are no symptoms of other psychiatric conditions, no clouding of consciousness, and no hallucinations in other modalities.

• **Olfactory Hallucinations** are far less common than the auditory or visual types, and their presence (along with gustatory and tactile hallucinations) warrants a medical investigation. These hallucinations can occur in:

> • Patients with psychotic disorders
> • Patients with coexisting psychiatric disorders and epilepsy
> • Patients with comorbid psychiatric and medical problems

Unfortunately, olfactory hallucinations rarely involve fragrances like rose petals. The most common smells are described as burning rubber, rotting garbage or very strong body odors. These smells often are of personal relevance to patients. Smell is the sense most closely linked to memory, and these hallucinations are often accompanied by strong feelings. The olfactory association areas are in the frontal lobes and limbic system (hypothalamus and amygdala).

Olfactory hallucinations accompany hallucinations in other modalities, as well as delusions. For example, patients with somatic delusions ("I'm rotting inside") may have accompanying olfactory hallucinations. Paranoid patients who believe they are being subjected to poisonous gases can hallucinate the smell of a noxious substance being piped in through their heating or air-conditioning vents.

• **Gustatory Hallucinations** involve more than just having unusual sense of taste in matters. These are the least common type and occur in the same group of conditions as do olfactory hallucinations. Patients who believe they are being poisoned may experience unusual tastes. Like olfactory hallucinations, these are rarely pleasant, often being described as metallic, acid, bitter or some bizarre combination of tastes. Psychotropic medication can have an effect on taste sensation. Lithium (metallic), zopiclone (metallic) and disulfiram (garlic-like) are common examples.

• **Somatic Hallucinations** are made up of three types:

1. Kinesthetic hallucinations are sensations of moving body parts such as joint position, body rotation, etc.

2. Cenesthetic or **visceral hallucinations** involve internal organs ("My spleen aligned itself along the axis of the equator")

3. Tactile hallucinations involve disorders of bodily sensation, such as:

formication — the sensation of insects crawling on the skin
haptic — the sensation of being touched
hygric — involves shifts in fluid ("All my lymph is in my head")
thermal — temperature related ("My ears are burning")

Like the other types of hallucinations, these are most common in psychotic conditions, temporal lobe epilepsy and migraine headaches. They are often paired with either **somatic delusions** or **delusions of control**. Because delusions are often based on a kernel of truth, psychotic patients may be describing actual perceptions in a distorted fashion.

Hypnagogic hallucinations occur while falling asleep, and **hypnopompic hallucinations** occur while awakening. These experiences occur in a large percentage of the population, and are not considered pathological by themselves. They can also occur during periods of illness where dehydration, fever or sedating medications are given. These hallucinations are usually visual, but can be auditory or tactile. While their duration is brief, they can occur as complex hallucinations. Hypnagogic and hypnopompic hallucinations occur in narcolepsy.

Many adults have had the experience of hearing their names called, only to find there was no one there. Other brief, familiar sounds (footsteps, doors closing, etc.) are also commonly experienced and are not pathological. **Bereavement** is the reaction to, and grieving process endured, after the death of a loved one. This period is often filled with "hallucinatory" experiences involving the deceased person.

(II) Illusions are *misperceptions* of existing stimuli. Actual percepts are exaggerated, distorted or altered so that they appear as something different to the person, but remain within the existing sensory modality (in other words, an object which is seen does not become transformed into a sound). Illusory experiences are affected by particular factors:

• The need to make sense of the environment; here, illusions "fill in the blanks" left by inattention or uncertainty; for example, misreading a word or being oblivious to a spelling mistake because the reader "knew what was meant" in the passage.

• Emotional state or expectation; a person who is frightened by walking alone at night is more likely to see a menacing figure in the shadows than if he were with someone else or walking the same route in daylight. **Pareidolia** refers to a type of imagery that persists when looking at a real object. The illusion and real stimulus exist simultaneously, but the pareidolic illusion is recognized as unreal. An example of this is seeing faces or shapes in clouds. Such illusions can be so striking that they require little imagination to visualize.

(III) Disturbances of Self and Environment
Depersonalization is a change in the perception of self, causing the individual to feel *as if* he or she has become unreal.

Derealization is a change in the awareness or the perception of the external world. It may be difficult to make a clear distinction between the two perceptions because patients may feel themselves blending into the surroundings during an episode of depersonalization. These conditions have the following associated features:

> • They are unpleasant, and cause anxiety or dysphoria
> • Patients retain an awareness that their experience is unreal (as opposed to dissociation)
> • Typical descriptions involve leaving one's body or somehow being outside of one's self; "looking down at myself from the ceiling" or "watching myself in a movie" are common descriptions of experiences

A theme of inadequacy is frequently reported. Patients feel as if they have become barren, deficient or incompetent. Often there is a distortion of time, which can seem either accelerated or slowed down. These experiences are common among psychologically healthy people.

(IV) Disturbances of Quality or Size

Micropsia is the perception of seeing things as being smaller than their actual size. **Macropsia** is the perception of objects seeming larger than their actual size.

Dysmegalopsia is the perception of seeing one side of an object as being larger than the other (something like the faces in a Picasso painting).

(V) Disturbances in the Intensity of Perception

In these alterations, sensory input is either augmented or diminished in intensity. For example, **hyperacusis** occurs when sounds are experienced as louder than they actually are. Smell, touch, taste, and sight (called **visual hyperesthesia** when enhanced) can all be similarly affected.

(VI) Disturbances of Experience

Déjà vu is a French term meaning "already seen" or "there's nothing new in that." It is used to denote a feeling of familiarity to situations that are novel. **Jamais vu**, meaning "never seen," is applied to situations that are familiar but strike the person as something they have not experienced.

These phenomena occur in people without mental illnesses and in a variety of medical and psychiatric disorders. The most common organic cause is temporal lobe epilepsy. Schizophrenia is the psychiatric diagnosis most often associated with frequent or severe experiences of this kind. When pathological, these disturbances are called **identifying paramnesias**. They can cause difficulty with the veracity of memory. Patients may not be able to accurately recall if an event occurred or not (as if it may have happened in a dream and the person can't be certain). Time perception can also be altered. Patients experiencing déjà vu may think that little or no time has passed because experiences seem familiar to them.

An **autoscopic hallucination** refers to the experience of seeing oneself as if in a mirror image, or projected onto the external world. Recognition is intact, and the image is correctly identified by the person. The opposite can also occur, called **negative autoscopy** or **heautoscopy**. Here, the person looks in the mirror and sees nothing. These conditions can be a feature of parietal lobe lesions which can also cause other abnormalities of perception:

> • **Anosognosia** — unawareness of physical illness, or nonrecognition of one side of the body (hemi-inattention)
> • **Prosopagnosia** — the inability to recognize familiar faces

Pseudohallucinations

Pseudohallucinations retain the quality of a perception without a stimulus; however, the person recognizes that the perceived event is not actually occurring. True hallucinations appear to be concrete, real, and happening apart from the patient (in their **external** or **objective space**). Pseudohallucinations occur in subjective, inner space. Patients refer to the "inner eye" or "inner ear" as perceiving the stimulus, which is usually auditory or visual. Pseudohallucinations can be vivid and formed. The "pseudo" part refers to preserved insight on the patient's part; it does not refer to poorly formed perceptions (called **elementary hallucinations**). In other words, these experiences are "pseudo" because there is an awareness of their false origin, not because of vague stimuli. In these situations, the patient's **reality perception** is impaired, but **reality testing** remains intact.

How Do I Ask About Perceptual Disorders?

Perceptual disturbances, along with disorders of thought content, are usually the most difficult to ask about in interviews.

There is an understanding among the lay population that lusions and hallucinations make one "crazy," and som tients become offended by questions in these areas.

In some cases, behavior is altered because patients are responding to hallucinations (e.g. being distracted by having to pay attention to the interviewer's voice while simultaneously experiencing hallucinations). In other situations, patients simply won't share their experiences, or have command hallucinations telling them to say nothing to interviewers!

When asking about perceptual disturbances, indicate you know they occur and that you are prepared to discuss them:

• *"Mr. Domi, a lot of people with difficulties like yours have some other symptoms as well. In order to be thorough, I'd like to ask you about some of these things so I have a complete understanding of what's been happening."*
• *"Have you had any unusual experiences?"*
• *"Have things been happening around you that seem puzzling or don't make sense?"*

One of the distinguishing features of hallucinations is that they seem as real as actual perceptions. A key point in establishing this is the **lack of corroboration** (i.e. other people around the patient do not share the experience). After asking the above questions, patients either share their experiences, or will ask you to be more specific about what you mean:

• *"Have you heard a voice from someone not in the room?"*
• *"Have you seen something that others couldn't see?"*
• *"Have you had experiences such as . . . (example of a hallucination) that others didn't share?"*

If the presence of any perceptual abnormality can be established, treat this as you would any other symptom and get as much detail as possible. Questions should assess duration, quality, intensity, variation, associated events, etc.

- *"Did you recognize whose voice it was?"*
- *"Did the voice/voices tell you to do something?"*
- *"Did you comply? Why or why not?"*

The question, *"Did the voice seem to come from inside or outside your head?"* is often asked. The significance of this is that true auditory hallucinations are considered to originate outside the self, e.g. from radio towers. However, true hallucinations can also be perceived as coming from within.

Another way of asking this question is to inquire whether the experience felt like a product of the person's mind (i.e. as are obsessions) or whether it was a completely external experience. Other questions can be posed as follows:

- *"Have you ever experienced a taste that wasn't due to something you were eating?"*

- *"Have you smelled something that didn't fit with the situation you were in at the time?"*

- *"Have you ever experienced a strong/bad taste or smell that you couldn't account for?"*

- *"Have you had sensations in your body that felt like they were due to unseen forces?"* (e.g. being touched or moved by something, ants crawling on your skin, internal organs being shifted, etc.)

10/ Insight, Judgment & Cognitive Functioning

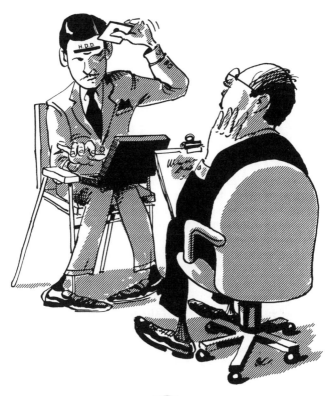

What Factors Determine Insight & Judgment?

Insight refers to the knowledge and awareness of the parameters involved in an event, process or decision. In mental health, this term is used to describe:

- An awareness of having an illness
- An understanding of the factors contributing to the illness
- An appreciation that various signs and symptoms are part of a disease process

Judgment is the opinion or conclusion arrived at by a patient, and generally refers to:

- A decision
- Whether or not a certain action took place, and why
- Weighing the consequences of doing or not doing something

Insight is a *cognitive awareness*, and is technically a component of thought content. Judgment involves both a *cognitive awareness* (decision) and an *action* (behavior). Intact insight and judgment are the end result of many factors: intelligence, accurate perception (of both internal and external events), absence of significant mood states, the ability to understand and communicate ideas, intact cognitive abilities, impulse control, and capacity for abstract thinking. Insight and judgment are crucial factors in determining the success of therapeutic interventions and the patient's prognosis.

How Is the Degree of Insight Determined?

Because insight occurs along a continuum, there are three levels or degrees that are used to describe the awareness patients have of their illnesses.

Full Insight
- Recognizes that signs and symptoms are part of an illness
- Understands that treatment may involve changing lifestyle
- Cooperates fully with treatment initiatives

Partial Insight
- Recognizes that there are problems, but does not attribute them to an illness
- May understand that others see them as ill
- Variable ability to modify behavior and accept treatment

Impaired Insight
- Denies having an illness or that there are problems
- Has no capacity to understand the concerns of others
- Poor compliance with treatment

How Is Judgment Determined?

Judgment is a process that leads to a decision or an action. In interview situations, this is an assessment of what the person did or didn't do with respect to his or her illness. Judgment can be determined using the following criteria:

- Ability to enumerate the pros & cons for a course of action
- The degree to which actions benefit the patient
- The extent to which insight is present
- The degree of contemplation prior to taking action

Poor judgment is evidenced when patients engage in activities with a high probability for damaging consequences (regardless of how impulsively they were carried out):

- Shoplifting
- Buying sprees
- Physical assault
- Promiscuity
- Reckless driving
- Vandalism

How Is Cognitive Functioning Tested?

The areas tested in the MSE as part of a comprehensive interview are:

- **Orientation** (Section I)
- **Attention & Concentration** (II)
- **Memory** (III)
  - Registration/Immediate
  - Short-Term/Recent
  - Long-Term/Remote
- **Intelligence Estimation** (IV)
- **Knowledge Base/Fund of Information** (V)
- **Capacity to Read and Write** (VI)
- **Abstraction/Concrete Thinking** (VII)
- **Visuospatial Ability** (VIII)

(I) Orientation is tested according to the following:
- *Time* (time of day, day of week, date, month, year, season)
- *Place* (hospital/clinic/office address & floor level, town or city, state, county, country)
- *Person* (identity of the person and recognition of family members, friends, health care providers, etc.)

Orientation is usually lost in the sequence of:
time (most common) > place > person (least common)

(II) Attention & Concentration
Attention is the ability to direct mental energy when fully alert. It is a conscious, willful focusing of cognitive processes while excluding competing stimuli (such as mood state, thoughts, perceptions, etc.). **Concentration** is the sustained focus of attention for a period of time.

Attention is assessed by checking the person's **digit span** (the number of numbers they can recall both forward and backward). You can usually start by testing 4 numbers recited in a forward fashion. Most adults have digit recall spans of between 5 to 7 numbers forward and 4 to 6 numbers backward, without errors, and completed within 30 seconds. Read off the numbers so that there are pauses of about one second between them. Avoid adding emphasis to the numbers as you read them. Numbers that are grouped too closely or with some rhythm can give a spuriously good result. For example, many companies have developed a jingle so that their phone numbers are more memorable. Another consideration is to avoid using numbers in a sequence (5-6-7-8) or exclusively odd/even numbers.

Concentration is most frequently tested with **serial seven subtractions**. Patients are not allowed to use any aid in this test, including their fingers. You can introduce this as follows, "I'd like you to start with the number 100 and subtract 7; then, from this number, subtract 7 and keep going." Alternative numerical tests are:

- Subtracting serial 3's starting at 20
- Serial additions
- Starting at another number using a different interval of subtraction (e.g. 103 minus 8)

(III) Memory
Registration is the instantaneous recall of new information; this is also called **immediate memory**, and is dependent on alertness and adequate concentration.

Short-term memory is thought to have a capacity for about 7 items over 20 seconds, though this can be increased with training; **recent memory** is sometimes used synonymously, but is also used to denote events that occurred in the past few hours. Depending on intact processes, this information is either discarded or committed to long-term memory.

Long-term memory has no demonstrable limits of storage and provides the **fund of knowledge** for patients; this is also called **remote memory** or **delayed recall**; this type of memory remains quite stable over time.

The most common test of verbal memory involves word re-call. This is used to test **immediate memory** (registration) and **short-term memory** (recent memory). The patient is given a list of three to five words and asked to recall them after about five minutes. The words chosen should have the following characteristics:

> • They should be unrelated to each other
> • They should not be something in the room or that is shown to the patient
> • They should be unrelated to the person's vocation or interests (e.g. don't ask an auto mechanic to re member a lug nut, cam shaft, and exhaust manifold)

Other tests of short-term memory are:

> • A name, address and zip code of a fictitious person
> • A short "story" of three to four sentences having about 25 points of information; an intact response involves remembering in the vicinity of 15 details
> • Word lists of about 15 items which can be related or unrelated; intact recall is considered to be some where in the vicinity of 50% of the words which de-clines as age increases

If a patient cannot remember all of the items, it is a common practice to prompt them. This can be done initially by stating the category of the missing item(s) (e.g. Was it a color? . . . A brand of soap?). If this doesn't work, present a list of other words which include the missing item(s). This provides patients with more help than listing the category. Failing this prompt may indicate a more serious impairment. Make sure you don't mention the missing item too close to the beginning of the list, and don't add any inflection to your voice for the correct word. There is no established standard with which to assess performance of short-term memory. If the patient requires prompting or a word list, record this as such.

Short-term memory can also be assessed by using **visual design reproduction tests**. One such test involves copying a design from memory that was placed in front of the patient for 30 seconds. These designs are usually an amalgamation of several geometric shapes.

Long-term memory can be assessed in terms of recent events (hours to days) or remote events (years). This can be tested in a practical manner in interviews by giving patients questions to which you can verify the answer. For example, the following information is usually readily available:

- Date of birth
- Address, zip code, and phone number
- Previous appointments or hospitalizations
- Medication type and dosage
- Recollection of your name (if you gave it)

(IV) Intelligence involves:

- The assimilation and recall of factual information
- Logical reasoning and problem-solving skills
- Abstraction, generalization, and symbolization

Intelligence can be gauged in interviews by:

- Degree of insight, judgment and abstract thinking
- Fund of knowledge

- Vocabulary (considered the best single indicator)
- Level of education, vocation, interests & hobbies

Three distinct types of intelligence have been described: mechanical, abstract, and social. Intelligence is usually reported as an **intelligence quotient (I.Q.)**

$$I.Q. = \frac{mental\ age}{chronological\ age} \times 100$$

Mental age is a measure of intellectual level. The most widely used and best standardized intelligence test is the Wechsler Adult Intelligence Scale (WAIS). The current version is the **WAIS-R** (R for revised). Because chronological age has such a bearing on IQ, there are separate versions for schoolchildren (ages 5 to 15) and preschoolers (ages 4 to 6). By definition, a normal IQ is 100, and mental retardation is defined as an IQ less than 70. Superior intelligence is above 120.

(V) Knowledge base can be estimated by incidental factors during the interview or may need to be more fully explored if cognitive deficits are discovered in other areas of testing. Head injuries and dementia are the most common causes of permanent knowledge deficits. The pseudodementia of depression can give the appearance of impaired cognitive functioning because patients tend to answer with *"I don't know"* responses. When pressed to respond, they often can, if sufficient time is allowed. Common questions involve:

- Naming political figures
- Significant dates (e.g. World War I or II)
- Capital cities, neighboring states, etc.

This information is "common knowledge" and doesn't have to involve the personal significance of the questions used to test remote memory.

(VI) Capacity to Read and Write

Assessment of these basic functions is often omitted in initial interviews. Illiteracy is present at an unfortunately high rate, and can be masked by people with good verbal skills. It is common for illiterate patients to be able to sign their names, which is often all that is required in clinical settings. Having patients write down their names and the date and (later) follow a simple written command screens for deficits. It is also useful to have patients write a sentence on the page.

(VII) Abstraction/Concrete Thinking

Abstract thinking is a complex mental ability. It requires the ability to think in a multidimensional manner by keeping all the characteristics of a "mental set" in mind and integrating the nuances into a new understanding. In interviews, patients demonstrate abstract thinking when they can appreciate all the meanings of an item, list similarities and differences, use logical reasoning, and grasp the "whole picture."

The opposite of abstraction is **concrete thinking**. This is a literal, unimaginative, narrow understanding of a concept. It is also called **one-dimensional thinking** and is often a feature of lower intelligence. Examples are as follows:

• Whiskey kills more people than bullets.
abstract — alcohol is deadlier to more people than gunfire
concrete — bullets don't drink

Abstract/Concrete Thinking can be tested with:

• **Similarities & Differences**   • **Proverbs**

The **similarities test** involves comparing two objects and listing common qualities. For example, *"What are the similarities between a chair and a desk?"*

abstract — both furniture, things can be put on them, etc.
concrete — four legs, made of wood, touch the floor, etc.

Abstraction involves function instead of form and the ability to generalize from particulars. The **differences test** requires patients to consider similar objects and list their distinguishing features (e.g. wine goblet vs. coffee mug)

Proverb interpretation is another commonly used method to test abstraction. Proverbs are "common truths" or generalizations born of experience. A concrete interpretation misses the "spirit" or message contained in the saying:

• The golden hammer opens an iron door.
abstract — the right touch is all that is needed
concrete — you'd have to hit it awfully hard!

Some clinicians do not consider proverbs a good test of abstraction because they are too culturally specific.

(VIII) Visuospatial Functions
This is tested in the MSE by assessing **constructional ability**. Patients are asked to draw a figure (usually geometric) on a piece of paper. The **Mini-Mental State Examination (MMSE)** uses interlocking pentagons for this test. The aspects involved in scoring the drawing are preserving: (i) the sides, (ii) the angles & (iii) interlocking corners. Another common test is to have patients draw a cube showing the correct three-dimensional orientation.

The **clock drawing test** has been used. Patients are asked to draw a complete clock face and indicate a certain time. Drawings are scored for: completeness (all the numbers), correctness (numbers in the proper place and sequence) and orientation (numbers on both sides and evenly spaced).

Examples of MSE Reports
Example 1

M.E. is a 29-year-old college student brought to the hospital by her roommate. Despite having final exams, M.E. had been busying herself with a wide number of activities unrelated to her studies.

Ms. M. E.'s **appearance** was that of a woman who looks her stated age and is dressed in mismatched clothes, consisting of a suit jacket, leotards and hiking boots. In the interview, her **behavior** involved refusing to be seated, and speaking only if she was allowed to walk around the room. She rummaged through her purse at the beginning of the interview and then wrote out several lists for the remainder of the time. She was superficially **cooperative** with the assessment and said she'd talk as long as she could make her lists and if the interview didn't last more than ten minutes. She was considered **reliable**, but biased towards minimizing the details of her activities.

Her **speech** was loud, rapid and pressured, but remained understandable and had proper syntax. Prosody was exaggerated, regardless of the content. **Thought process** involved connections that were generally logical. On two occasions she was unable to repeat the questions posed to her or to relate the connection between them and what she was just saying. The **content** of her thoughts had to do with her plans to start at a senior management level in the Fortune 500 company of her choice after graduation. She had developed powerful insights into the business world, and even offered the interviewer an autographed copy of her term paper.

Her **affect** was forceful and exuberant, and remained consistently high during the interview. She described her mood as energetic and that she'd never felt better. She gave her mood a score of nine out of ten (she says she'll be a ten after graduation). She denied any **perceptual** problems. She stated she felt well and couldn't see why others were concerned. On this basis, her **insight** and **judgment** were both deemed to be impaired.

Testing of her **cognitive functions** revealed that she was completely oriented. She was able to **register** four items and **recalled** them at around five minutes. However, she could not recite the interviewer's name or her exam schedule, so her **long-term memory** was considered impaired. Her attention and concentration were intact for six numbers forward and four backward. She performed three **serial subtractions** correctly and then told a story about the number seventy-nine. She was able to enumerate a considerable list of **similarities and differences**, many of which demonstrated a high level of abstraction. Her **knowledge base** was consistent with her level of education and her **intelligence** seemed to be above average.

Example 2

Mrs. D.E. is a 47-year-old separated woman who is employed as a professional cello player. After missing her third rehearsal, she was brought to the clinic after being found in the basement of her home.

• Her appearance is that of a woman appearing older than her age. She was dressed in a housecoat and slippers. She is thin, has an odor of poor hygiene, and has old scars visible on her left wrist and forearm.

• She sat throughout the interview in an immobile position with her hands at her sides and her head slumped forward on her chest. She made no spontaneous movements when speaking.

• She was uncooperative with the interview and said she wanted to be left alone. The information she shared did not seem reliable.

• Her speech was fluent and syntactically correct. There was a latency of several seconds before replying to questions. She spoke in a monotonous manner with no variability or prosody.

• Her thought process showed intermittent loosening of associations with periods of rambling when she was asked open-ended questions.

• Her thought content involved delusions of persecution and being infested. On a recent trip overseas, she inadvertently knocked over the display of a merchant who was selling rare cultural artifacts. This merchant put a "curse" on her. Mrs. D.E. has been coping poorly and declining since that time. She is convinced she has some type of flesh-eating organism inside her.

• She has passive wishes to die, but denies that she'd do anything to harm herself. There are no thoughts of wanting to harm others.

• Her affect was flat and showed no range during the interview. She felt doomed and hopeless, and described her mood as depressed.

• She described perceptual abnormalities in the form of tactile (beetles crawling on her skin) and cenesthetic hallucinations (the lining of her intestines was being gnawed away). She was also constantly harassed by the voice of the merchant she met while on her overseas trip.

• Her insight and judgment were both considered impaired on the basis of the bizarre delusions, her inability to understand that she is ill, and because she needed others to bring her in for help.

• Cognitive testing revealed that she was only oriented to person, month, year and season. She knew she was in a hospital, but not which one. She was able to register only one object after two tries, and was not able to recall this object after three minutes' time. Digit span was intact only for three numbers forwards and two numbers backwards. She did not attempt the serial sevens test. She was able to follow a written command and wrote a sentence ("I am going to die for what I did."). In response to many questions she replied, "I don't know." Testing of similarities and differences revealed concrete thinking and highly idiosyncratic replies.

References

American Psychiatric Association
Practice Guidelines: Psychiatric Evaluation of Adults
American Psychiatric Association, Washington D.C., 1996

American Psychiatric Association
Diagnostic & Statistical Manual of Mental Disorders, 4th Edition
American Psychiatric Association, Washington D.C., 1994

N. Andreason & D. Black
Introductory Textbook of Psychiatry, 2nd Edition
American Psychiatric Press, Inc., Washington, D.C., 1995

R. Campbell
Psychiatric Dictionary, 7th Edition
Oxford University Press, New York, 1996

A. C. Doyle
The Complete Sherlock Holmes, Vol.1, p. 352
Doubleday & Co. Inc., New York

H. Kaplan, B. Sadock, & J. Grebb, Editors
Synopsis of Psychiatry, 8th Edition
Williams & Wilkins, Baltimore, 1998

D. Kaufman
Clinical Neurology for Psychiatrists, 4th Edition
W. B. Saunders Co., Philadelphia, 1995

J. Morrison & R. Muñoz
Boarding Time, 2nd Edition
American Psychiatric Press Inc., Washington, D.C., 1996

D. O'Neill
Brain Stethoscopes: The Use and Abuse of Brief Mental Status Schedules
Postgraduate Medical Journal (69), p. 599-601, Aug. 1993

E. Othmer & S. Othmer
The Clinical Interview Using DSM-IV, Volume 1: The Fundamentals
American Psychiatric Press Inc., Washington D.C., 1994

R. Rogers
Clinical Assessment of Malingering and Deception
The Guilford Press, New York, 1988

A. Sims
Symptoms in the Mind, 2nd Edition
Saunders, London, England, 1995

M. Taylor
The Neuropsychiatric Mental Status Exam
PMA Publishing Corp., New York, 1981

E. Zuckerman
The Clinician's Thesaurus, 4th Edition
Clinician's Toolbox, The Guilford Press, New York, 1995

Index

The Author

Dave Robinson is a psychiatrist practicing in London, Ontario, Canada. His particular interests are consultation-liaison psychiatry, undergraduate and post-graduate education. He is a graduate of the University of Toronto Medical School and is a Lecturer in the Department of Psychiatry at the University of Western Ontario in London, Canada.

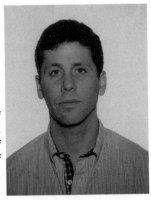

The Artist

Brian Chapman is a resident of Oakville, Ontario, Canada. He was born in Sussex, England and moved to Canada in 1957. Brian was formerly a Creative Director at Mediacom. He continues to freelance and is versatile in a wide range of media. He is a master of the caricature, and his talents are constantly in demand.

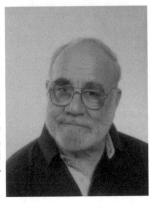

Rapid Psychler Press

Rapid Psychler Press was founded in 1994 with the aim of producing textbooks and resource materials that further the use of humor in mental health education. In addition to textbooks, Rapid Psychler Press specializes in producing slides and overheads for presentations.